Learni... ...*e*

ELDERL . ᴇOPLE

Linda Thomas
SRN

Nurse Adviser, Royal College of
Nursing Society of Geriatric
Nursing

HODDER AND STOUGHTON
LONDON SYDNEY AUCKLAND TORONTO

LEARNING TO CARE SERIES

General Editors

JEAN HEATH, BA, SRN, SCM, CERT ED
National Health Learning Resources Unit, Sheffield
City Polytechnic

SUSAN E NORMAN, SRN, NDNCERT, RNT
Senior Tutor, The Nightingale School, West Lam-
beth Health Authority

Titles in this series include:

Learning to Care on the Medical Ward
A MATTHEWS
Learning to Care in the Community
P TURTON and J ORR
Learning to Care on the ENT Ward
D STOKES

British Library Cataloguing in Publication Data
Thomas, Linda L.
  Learning to care for elderly people. –
  (Learning to care)
  1. Geriatric nursing
  I. Title   II. Series
  610.73'65   RC954

  ISBN 0 340 37063 7

First published 1985
Copyright © 1985 L. Thomas
Third impression 1987

Typeset in 10/11 pt Trump Medieval by
Rowland Phototypesetting Ltd, Bury St Edmunds, Suffolk

Printed in Great Britain for
Hodder and Stoughton Educational,
a division of Hodder and Stoughton Ltd,
Mill Road, Dunton Green, Sevenoaks, Kent, by
Richard Clay Ltd, Bungay, Suffolk.

EDITORS' FOREWORD

In most professions there is a traditional gulf between theory and its practice, and nursing is no exception. The gulf is perpetuated when theory is taught in a theoretical setting and practice is taught by the practitioner.

This inherent gulf has to be bridged by students of nursing and publication of this series is an attempt to aid such bridge building.

It aims to help relate theory and practice in a meaningful way whilst underlining the importance of the person being cared for.

It aims to introduce students of nursing to some of the more common problems found in each new area of experience in which they will be asked to work.

It aims to de-mystify some of the technical language they will hear, putting it in context, giving it meaning and enabling understanding.

PREFACE

When I first entered the field of geriatric nursing, books on the subject were few and far between. It has been a great personal pleasure to see the numbers of specialist textbooks increase, mirroring the growing interest in this fascinating and challenging specialty.

This book is intended as an introduction to the care of the elderly for learners entering the Department of Geriatric Medicine for the first time. I hope that it will serve to allay some of their fears, give them a basic understanding of how the department functions and above all help them to understand and meet the needs of their elderly clients.

We all have a vested interest in ensuring that standards of care for elderly people continue to improve. To that end, I hope that the learners who read this book will be encouraged to find out more about the specialty.

In writing it, I have drawn very heavily on my own experiences and observations. It would be impossible to name individually all the people who have influenced my career in the care of the elderly. Suffice to say that without them, there would have been no book.

Finally, thanks are due to the gentle and persuasive publishing team for their continued encouragement and to my husband Stephen, sworn enemy of all procrastinators!

Linda Thomas

CONTENTS

Introduction

Misapprehensions about ageing abound. Disease and illness are accepted – even expected – as an inevitable part of the ageing process. Old people are seen as a pitiable burden who have outlived their usefulness to Society and who are a drain on scarce economic resources.

The Population Census taken on April 5th, 1981 revealed that while the size of the total population of Great Britain had grown by only about 0.6%, the number of pensioners (women aged 60 and over, men aged 65 and over) increased by about 10% to 9½ million.

Moreover, it is predicted that there will be a 40% increase in the number of people over the age of 75 and a 50% increase in those over 85 by the end of the century.

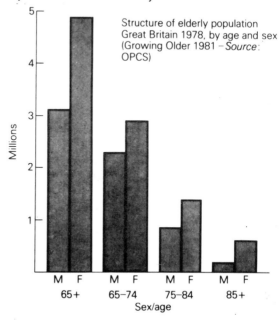

Structure of elderly population Great Britain 1978, by age and sex (Growing Older 1981 – *Source*: OPCS)

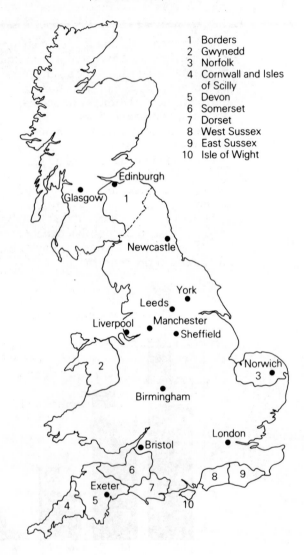

Counties with the highest proportion
of pensioners in 1981
(*Source*: OPCS)

1 Borders
2 Gwynedd
3 Norfolk
4 Cornwall and Isles
   of Scilly
5 Devon
6 Somerset
7 Dorset
8 West Sussex
9 East Sussex
10 Isle of Wight

Edinburgh
Glasgow
1
Newcastle
York
Leeds
Liverpool
Manchester
Sheffield
2
Norwich
3
Birmingham
London
Bristol
6
8 9
Exeter
7
5
10
4

Ageing and Society

Statistically speaking, the arbitrary arrival of old age comes with retirement. Many people choose to move away from familiar haunts and lifestyles, opting for a new way of life in attractive coastal resorts. For some, retirement will be happy and fulfilled; for others, the effects of retirement will be profoundly disturbing, leading to a sense of alienation and worthlessness.

Negative effects of retirement:

loss of income
loss of status
loss of purpose
loss of social contacts
depression
deterioration of health

The effects of a dramatically reduced income can severely restrict the way in which a retired person lives. Not only 'luxury' items are cut from the budget as worries about essential necessities such as food and heating begin to dominate.

Adequate preparation for retirement, perhaps in the form of gradual withdrawal from full-time work and with the help of pre-retirement classes, may go some way to offset the change from the discipline of work to the acquisition of unlimited leisure time.

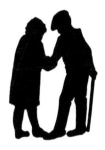

Positive aspects of retirement
More time – for: 'formal' and 'informal' education (Open University, University of the Third Age)

involvement in local politics
involvement in voluntary work

pursuing hobbies, learning new skills

involvement with the family

The Elderly in the Community

Only a very small proportion of the elderly population is ever in institutionalised care at any time – about 5–7% in total. Moreover, most elderly people live at home quite independently, requiring little if any help, and consider themselves to be in good health.

For those requiring some support, a succession of Government papers in the last few years (*A Happier Old Age*, 1978; *Growing Older*, 1981; *Care in the Community*, 1981) has reinforced the view that resources for care should be moved into the community.

While a range of statutory services is available, with increasing back-up support from voluntary agencies, it is also a fact that very many elderly people are supported by families, friends and neighbours.

Examples of voluntary and statutory domiciliary services:

Home Help
Meals on Wheels
Day Centres
Luncheon Clubs
Primary Health Care
Neighbourhood Care Groups
Day Hospitals

Most services are designed to support old people living alone. Statutory support for the network of 'informal carers' coping with elderly dependants is still inadequate, although recognition of a need for support is growing. For example, the provision of 'respite' or 'holiday relief' beds offering a short stay in hospital or in a Local Authority home to elderly dependants enables carers to have a break.

Health Care of the Elderly

Institutionalised care of the elderly has its roots in the appalling conditions of the nineteenth century workhouse infirmaries. The helpless and bedridden elderly sick were likely to be tended by pauper nurses scarcely fitter, younger or more able than their charges.

Pauper nurses were banned in 1897, but the care of the inmates had improved little when Dr Marjory Warren of the West Middlesex Hospital in London took charge of a workhouse infirmary in the 1930s.

A pioneer in improving the care of the elderly, she introduced the concept of rehabilitation and maintained that the elderly should have access to the same medical facilities as younger patients.

Developments in Geriatric Medicine

Geriatrics 'the medical care of the old'

from the Greek *geras* (old age), *iatreia* (treatment)

The term geriatric was first used in 1909 by Nascher

The association of geriatric medicine with chronic long-term care has gradually been overtaken by a more positive image. Consultant Geriatricians and Consultant Physicians with a special interest in Geriatric Medicine emphasise the necessity for dynamic treatment programmes for their elderly patients.

The philosophy of progressive patient care for the elderly is now a common factor everywhere despite the fact that many Departments of Geriatric Medicine are still housed in inadequate, converted buildings which bear little resemblance to the few purpose-built units which do exist.

The Department of Geriatric Medicine

Admission to Hospital

Admission to the Geriatric Unit may occur as a result of referral from various different agencies.

PATIENT
↓
referral by general practitioner
domiciliary visit by consultant geriatrician
accident and emergency department
day hospital
other hospital departments
↓
GERIATRIC DEPARTMENT

The acutely ill elderly person is likely to be admitted with multiple illnesses. Some degenerative changes are an inevitable part of the biological ageing process and some diseases are particularly prevalent in old age.

Geriatric admission wards should offer the same range of diagnostic procedures that are available to younger patients in general wards. It is always assumed initially that the patients' illnesses are treatable and their period in hospital temporary.

Routine tests:

temperature, pulse, respiration
blood pressure
chest X-ray
electrocardiograph
haematology/biochemistry
urinalysis

Rehabilitation

Having recovered from the acute phase of an illness, a longer period of rehabilitation may be necessary involving the skills of different members of the team.

The aim of rehabilitation should be to enable the patient to achieve a level of functional independence realistic to his needs. An integral part of the rehabilitation process is planning for discharge, whether to the patient's own home or to some kind of sheltered accommodation or institution. Effective communication with community services is therefore essential.

Occupational Therapist		Physio-therapist		Liaison Nurse		Community Psychiatric Nurse
Doctor		Chiropodist			Speech Therapist	
Family	Friends		Patient		Nurse	Social Worker
Chaplain		Primary Health Care Team		Social Services Department		Voluntary Services

Some members of the multidisciplinary team

Continuing Care

Some patients are never able to return home either to live independently or with support from others. There is a range of accommodation available to them according to the level of their capabilities:

sheltered housing/warden controlled accommodation
'part III' social services residential care home
private or voluntary residential care home or nursing home
National Health Service nursing home
continuing care ward in hospital

Nursing Care of the Elderly

Ageism – discriminative treatment of elderly people – is rife in modern society, where there is a tendency to value people according to their economic worth. The image of old people as a burden on health and social services, physically and mentally incapable and economically worthless, is prevalent.

More than any other age group, the elderly suffer from the effects of stereotyping. The term 'granny' immediately brings to mind a pink-cheeked old lady sitting cosily in front of a coal fire with her knitting. The term 'geriatric' is frequently used as one of abuse, not least by professional comedians, intimating absolute witlessness.

These attitudes have had an effect on the specialty of geriatric nursing. It is still sometimes erroneously viewed as a 'clinical backwater', requiring nothing more of its nurses than good basic nursing care and a strong back. The problems associated with the nursing care of the elderly have been well documented by two nurse researchers in particular, Doreen Norton and Thelma Wells.

Dynamic progressive patient care is a comparatively recent development. Historically, the geriatric specialty has been viewed as a 'dead-end' in career terms, especially for Registered Nurses. Student nurses have only been required to undertake practical experience in the specialty since 1979.

Because few tutorial staff had undergone training in geriatric care themselves prior to 1979, education has frequently lacked a positive approach. Nurses entering the specialty for the first time during their training may look forward to the experience with trepidation, expecting hard physical labour with little reward and no intellectual stimulation. The majority of them will be pleasantly

surprised to discover how much they enjoy the
challenge of caring for elderly people, and the
range of nursing skills they will be called upon
to use.

The Role of the Specialist Nurse

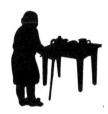

The role of the specialist nurse in the care of
the elderly differs according to the type of
environment in which she is working. The
needs of an acutely ill patient on an admission
ward are quite different to those of a client at
home with a long-standing health problem or a
patient in a continuing care ward in danger of
succumbing to the inertia of institutionalis-
ation. The means of planning care, however, is
a common factor:

Assessment of Need
Nursing Action Required
Implementation of Care
Evaluation of Care

On the whole, the pace on most wards specialising in the care of the elderly tends to be
less frenetic than that in, say, a busy surgical
ward. A tranquil atmosphere free from unnecessary clinical bustle where the atmosphere is relaxed and friendly is less alarming.

Maintaining Independence

Elderly patients in geriatric wards are no longer put to bed and kept there. On the contrary,
the most vital aspect in the care of an elderly
patient, and the most difficult to achieve, is
restoring and maintaining that patient's independence.

The easy option when confronted with an
elderly patient who has multiple disabilities is
to do everything for her. This short-term 'kind-
ness' will lead to long-term dependence.

The caring expert nurse will identify the means by which the patient can overcome disabilities. This requires in-depth physiological knowledge of the disabilities in question, awareness of available mechanical aids, the ability to liaise with other members of the team who are also working with the patient, and above all the skill and patience to ensure that the patient understands and is involved in the achievement of maximum functional independence.

Some significant dates in the development of the care of the elderly

1940   National Old People's Welfare Council founded (now known as Age Concern)

1948   Inaugural meeting of the Medical Society for the Care of the Elderly (now known as the British Geriatrics Society)

1962   Publication of *An Investigation of Geriatric Nursing Problems in Hospital* by Norton *et al*

1968   Publication of *Sans Everything* by Barbara Robb for the Aid for Elderly in Government Institutions (AEGIS) association

1973   Geriatric Nursing included in syllabus for student nurses as an option

        Joint Board of Clinical Nursing Studies produced curriculum for 6 month course on the care of the elderly and geriatric nursing (now under the auspices of the National Boards)

1975   Publication of *Improving Geriatric Care in Hospital* by the Royal College of Nursing and the British Geriatrics Society

1976   Royal College of Nursing Society of Geriatric Nursing founded

1979   All student nurses to undertake practical experience in geriatric nursing as a statutory requirement of their training

1980   Publication of *Problems in Geriatric Nursing Care* by Thelma Wells

1982   Doreen Norton appointed world's first Professor in Gerontological Nursing in Cleveland, Ohio

Working With the Team

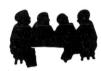

A bewildering number of health care professionals is involved in the day-to-day care of elderly patients. For ease of reference they are collectively referred to as 'the multidisciplinary team' and in most progressive Departments of Geriatric Medicine the team meets regularly to discuss the progress of patients at a case conference.

The contribution of the nurse at any discussion relating to patient care cannot be overestimated. Of all the members of the team, she is the one who has most contact with the patient and the patient's relatives and friends.

Honesty in reporting is vital – to hazard a guess about any aspect of a patient's progress when not absolutely certain of the facts could have a massive impact on plans for the patient's future.

Similarly, the specialist nurse needs to grasp the role of each member of the team very thoroughly in order to utilise all the available resources – how many nurses really understand the work of the chiropodist or social worker?

Nurses also need to ensure that every member of the team has agreed that they are working to the same end – pointless for the physiotherapist to help a patient relearn the skills of walking and climbing stairs if the nursing staff are taking the same patient everywhere in a wheelchair!

Post-basic courses:
Two post-basic courses are available for nurses on the care of the elderly, under the auspices of the National Boards. The short 22 day course (number 941) is intended for very experienced qualified staff. The longer 6 month course (number 298) for qualified staff gives an insight into the whole range of care of the elderly.

Effective Communication

Many elderly people feel their loss of status due to age and increasing frailty very keenly. It is very easy for nurses to adopt a patronising attitude towards their elderly patients, dubbing every female patient 'Gran' and every male patient 'Granddad' or 'Pops'.

Similarly, while some elderly people like to be known by their first names, others bitterly resent this uninvited familiarity. Effective communication by nurses begins with a genuine recognition of each patient as an individual.

In the face of humiliating incapacities – loss of speech following a stroke or shaming urinary incontinence, perhaps – many elderly patients are struggling to retain their identity and dignity. The ultimate indignity in these circumstances is to be scolded like a child. Caring for the elderly has *nothing* in common with caring for children.

Each incident of incontinence is far more shameful and embarrassing to the sufferer than it is distasteful for the nurse to deal with. Practical advice on the promotion of continence is now more widely available and a commonsense approach in the first instance will help to stave off a feeling of frustration and helplessness for both sufferer and nurse – is the toilet accessible or a commode conveniently to hand, can the patient get up from her chair, is her walking frame near her, can she manage her own clothing easily, is she wearing her own underwear?

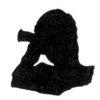

There are practical problems to be overcome in some instances when attempting to communicate effectively with elderly people. Nurses need to understand the operational intricacies of a variety of hearing aids, as well as ensuring that spectacles and dentures, if worn, are in place.

A gentle touch and simple, clear speech, particularly with blind or disorientated patients, are extremely effective means of communication. Shouting, arguing or adopting a superior patronising attitude with confused patients will only confuse them further. Try to imagine the bewilderment of the confused patient's mind, remember that any aggression is not directed at you personally, and it may remove your own apprehension in dealing with the patient.

Nursing in the Department of Geriatric Medicine

Not all old people are pleasant and easy to nurse; indeed, not all people are pleasant and easy to nurse. Recognition of an elderly person as an individual with unique needs is the first step to becoming a nurse skilled in the care of the elderly.

In the following chapters you will be introduced to some of the people you might come across when nursing the elderly sick in the Department of Geriatric Medicine.

TEST YOURSELF

Here are some points you might like to think about and discuss further:

1 Do you think the term 'geriatric' is always used in the right context?

2 Can you think of any examples of ageism – discriminatory treatment of the elderly – that you personally have come across?

3 Is there a local branch of the University of the Third Age in your area? Perhaps your Tutor might be prepared to invite one of its members to meet with your group.

4 What do you think are the main differences between nursing elderly patients in general wards and nursing elderly patients in Departments of Geriatric Medicine?

FURTHER READING

DHSS. 1983. *Elderly People in the Community: Their Service Needs.* London: HMSO.

MCFARLANE, BARONESS J. K. & CASTLEDINE, G. 1982. *A Guide to the Practice of Nursing Using the Nursing Process.* St. Louis: The C. V. Mosby Company.

NORTON, D., MCLAREN, R. & EXTON-SMITH, A. N. 1962. *An Investigation of Geriatric Nursing Problems in Hospital.* London: National Corporation for the Care of Old People. (Reprinted 1976, Churchill Livingstone.)

PHILLIPSON, C. 1982. *Capitalism and the Construction of Old Age.* London: The Macmillan Press Ltd.

ROSSITER, C. & WICKS, M. 1982. *Crisis or Challenge? Family Care, Elderly People and Social Policy.* London: Study Commission on the Family.

ROWLINGS, C. 1981. *Social Work with Elderly People.* London: George Allen and Unwin.

STOTT, M. 1981. *Ageing for Beginners – Understanding Everyday Experience.* Oxford: Basil Blackwell Publisher Ltd.

WELLS, T. J. 1980. *Problems in Geriatric Nursing Care.* Edinburgh: Churchill Livingstone.

YOUNG, P. (Ed). 1984. *Nursing the Aged.* Cambridge: Woodhead-Faulkner Ltd.

YURICK, A. G., SPIER, B. E., ROBB, S. S. & EBERT, N. J. 1984. *The Aged Person and the Nursing Process*, 2nd ed. Norwalk, Connecticut: Appleton-Century-Crofts.

2 Miss Smith who is admitted to the ward with congestive heart failure

HISTORY

Miss Smith is an 82 year old spinster living in a warden controlled flat. Although normally fairly active, she recently visited her G.P. as she had been suffering from occasional chest pains while out shopping.

Her G.P. arranges an appointment for her in a fortnight's time at the local hospital Out-patients' Department. In the meantime, Miss Smith finds she is becoming increasingly breathless while walking and notices that her ankles are swollen.

On the night before her appointment she sleeps restlessly in a chair, finding it difficult to breathe lying down. The Consultant Geriatrician examines her in the Geriatric Clinic of the Outpatients' Department and diagnoses *congestive cardiac failure.*

1 Blood enters right atrium via venae cavae
2 through tricuspid valve to right ventricle
3 leaves via pulmonary artery
4 to lung capillaries
5 to pulmonary veins
6 to left atrium
7 through mitral valve to left ventricle
8 to aorta and coronary arteries

The heart

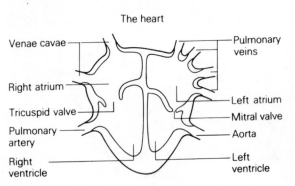

Cardiac failure

right ventricular failure (congestive cardiac failure)

right ventricle unable to match output into pulmonary artery with input from venous system leading to increased venous pressure

common causes in the elderly

left ventricular failure
lung disease (e.g. chronic bronchitis, emphysema)
congenital heart disease
mitral stenosis
myxoedema

left ventricular failure

left ventricle no longer able to pump blood into arterial system leading to lung congestion

common causes in the elderly
coronary artery disease
aortic stenosis
hypertension

The doctor suspects that Miss Smith may have underlying *ischaemic heart disease*. He arranges her admission to the Geriatric Unit as a matter of urgency.

Ischaemic heart disease:

The two coronary arteries supply the heart muscle (myocardium) with oxygen and nutrients.

1 Disease of the coronary arteries causes them to narrow (arteriosclerosis)
2 This reduces the blood supply to a part of the myocardium
3 This causes ischaemic heart disease

Ischaemia means: deficiency of blood

Congestive cardiac failure

Common signs and symptoms
dypsnoea
cyanosis
oedema of ankles
and sacrum
irregular rapid
pulse
cough
congestion of
jugular veins
enlarged liver
oliguria and
albuminuria

Miss Smith is very breathless and distressed when she arrives on the ward. Apart from feeling very ill, she was not expecting to be admitted to hospital and has nothing with her – no nightdress or toiletries and very little money. She is also very worried about letting the warden of her flat know where she is.

Two nurses quietly help her into bed, introducing themselves by name. One explains that anything Miss Smith needs in the way of food and toiletries and nightwear will be provided. Because she is so breathless, no attempt is made as yet to take a full nursing history. One nurse remains with Miss Smith while the doctor examines her and prescribes medical treatment.

While Miss Smith is being examined, the second nurse contacts her warden to explain what has happened and to find out a little about Miss Smith's personal circumstances.

Once the medical treatment has been prescribed to relieve her symptoms, a nursing care plan is devised identifying principal nursing needs and the best means of meeting them.

Medical treatment:

diuretic: to increase urinary output and relieve congestion
potassium supplement: to replace depletion caused by diuretic
digoxin therapy: to slow and strengthen the heartbeat
oxygen intermittently: to relieve dypsnoea
aminophylline: to relieve dypsnoea
morphine: to relieve pain

NURSING
CARE

Initial stages

As Miss Smith finds great difficulty in breathing while lying down (orthopnoea) she is nursed in an upright position with her head and back well supported with pillows. She is a thin, frail lady found to be at great risk from developing pressure sores.

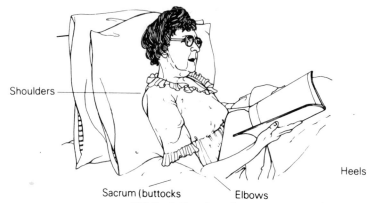

Susceptible pressure areas

Shoulders

Heels

Sacrum (buttocks   Elbows

While Miss Smith is encouraged to change position to relieve pressure, in practical terms this is very difficult at first because of her extreme breathlessness. A ripple mattress and bed cradle are used as mechanical aids to relieve pressure.

Although initially she is nursed in bed for the first few hours of her admission, she is encouraged to sit out in a chair on her second day in the ward. She finds this more comfortable with her back and head well supported and her legs supported and elevated. She prefers to sleep in the chair at night.

Particular care is taken to ensure that Miss Smith's pressure areas are relieved when she is sitting in the chair as she is just as much at risk from developing pressure sores as she would be if she were bedfast.

A commode is left within easy reach. Diuretic therapy, though dramatically improving her condition, could cause her untold misery if she has difficulty in reaching the toilet quickly. During the initial stages of her illness she needs considerable nursing help as any undue exertion causes breathlessness.

Her appetite is poor and she feels nauseated at first. Care is taken to ensure that she drinks enough fluid as she could become quickly dehydrated due to the diuretic therapy. Her intake and output of fluid is recorded on a fluid balance chart.

Her diet is an important factor in her nursing care. She needs light easily digested food attractively presented and a variety of choice of drinks. Monotonous offerings of minced meat, milk pudding and diluted orange squash will not tempt her appetite.

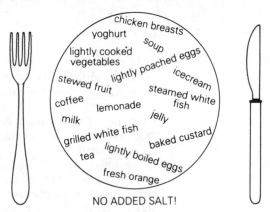

chicken breasts
yoghurt
soup
lightly cooked vegetables
lightly poached eggs
stewed fruit
icecream
steamed white fish
coffee
lemonade
milk
jelly
grilled white fish
baked custard
tea
lightly boiled eggs
fresh orange

NO ADDED SALT!

Rehabilitation

Miss Smith responds well to treatment and is gradually able to walk a little further every day. At first she finds it helpful to support herself with a Zimmer walking frame which has been supplied by the physiotherapist who has ensured that Miss Smith has the correct size of frame.

Initially Miss Smith needs the security of knowing someone is at her side when she is walking and that a chair will be readily available if she has an attack of breathlessness.

The warden of the flat visits Miss Smith soon after her admission, bringing her clothes and some personal belongings. As Miss Smith has neither close friends nor relatives, the medical social worker meets with Miss Smith and the warden to ascertain that all will be well should the multidisciplinary team decide to discharge her.

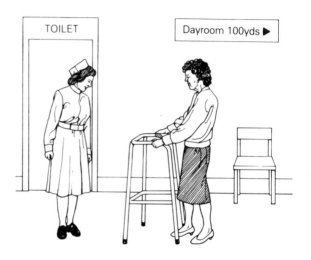

Planning discharge

At a group discussion involving members of the team who have been caring for Miss Smith, the decision is made to discharge Miss Smith to her sheltered accommodation following a stay in hospital of three weeks. It is agreed that the Geriatric Liaison Nurse will visit her one week after her discharge to check on her progress.

Although the warden of her flat will be available in an emergency, she is not able to offer practical support and so Meals-on-Wheels are ordered for Miss Smith and a home help to deal with the cleaning.

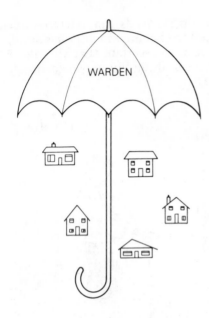

WARDEN

Age Concern describe sheltered accommodation as 'grouped housing for men and women normally over pensionable age where a resident Warden is employed and where convenient, well-planned self-contained dwellings for elderly people offer them the opportunity of retaining their independence yet giving security, the background support of a warden, and help in an emergency' (Age Concern, 1975).

CARE FOLLOWING DISCHARGE

It is intended that after leaving hospital, Miss Smith will continue with a small maintenance dose of digoxin, a diuretic and potassium supplement. A letter is sent to her G.P. immediately on her discharge informing him of her return home and of the treatment she has received and is still receiving.

Digoxin:
signs and symptoms of digoxin toxicity
nausea
cardiac
arrhythmias
confusion
vomiting
anorexia

usual maintenance dose in the elderly:
0.0625–0.125mg

As it is very important that Miss Smith understands the need for continuing with her medication, a nurse takes time to explain exactly when Miss Smith should take the tablets. She also stresses that any tablets at home which had been previously prescribed should be destroyed by flushing them down the toilet.

An appointment is made for Miss Smith to attend the Outpatients' Clinic in two weeks' time and an ambulance booked to ferry her there and back.

Check with your Tutor or Ward Sister that you understand the questions and have answered them fully.

1 If a patient is receiving diuretic therapy, what *environmental* influences could cause incontinence?

2 What do you think of the concept of 'sheltered accommodation'? List the advantages and disadvantages of a group of elderly people living together in this way. Have you ever visited any sheltered accommodation?

3 Name a voluntary organisation principally concerned with the care of the elderly. Is there a branch of this organisation in your area? Describe one of the schemes they have set up to help the elderly locally.

4 How do you recognise digoxin toxicity? If a patient is admitted to your ward described as suffering from the effects of 'polypharmacy', what would this mean to you? How could you as a nurse prevent this from happening again?

FURTHER
READING

AGE CONCERN. 1975. *Role of the Warden in Grouped Housing.* Mitcham, Surrey: Age Concern.
BEAUMONT, R. & KEANE, M. 1981. *Nursing Elderly Patients.* Key Facts Cards. Eastbourne, Sussex: Baillière Tindall.
IRVINE, R., BAGNALL, M. & SMITH, B. 1980. *The Older Patient – An Introduction to Geriatrics.* Sevenoaks: Hodder and Stoughton.
ROYAL COLLEGE OF PHYSICIANS. 1983. *Medication and the Elderly – a Report.* London: Royal College of Physicians.
WILCOCK, G. & MIDDLETON, A. 1984. *Geriatrics Pocket Consultant.* Oxford: Blackwell Scientific.

3

Mrs Jones who is admitted to the ward suffering from a cerebro-vascular accident (CVA or stroke)

Mrs Jones is a 79 year old widow who lives alone in a ground floor flat. Her daughter, who is 60, calls in to see her twice a week and on visiting one morning finds her mother on the floor beside the bed in her nightdress. She has been incontinent of urine and is too upset and dazed to say what has happened.

Her daughter calls an ambulance and Mrs Jones is taken to the nearest Casualty Department. A doctor diagnoses her as having suffered a *cerebro-vascular accident* with a *left hemiparesis*. Admission to the assessment and rehabilitation ward of the Geriatric Unit is arranged. Mrs Jones is accompanied by her daughter to the ward.

What is a cerebro-vascular accident?
The World Health Organisation has described a stroke (cerebro-vascular accident) as being 'due to a local disturbance in the blood supply to the brain; its onset is usually abrupt but may extend over a few hours or longer' (WHO, 1971).

The Circle of Willis – Cerebral Circulation
(blood supply to the brain)

Incidence of CVAs:

estimated 100,000 new strokes annually
75% over 65 years old

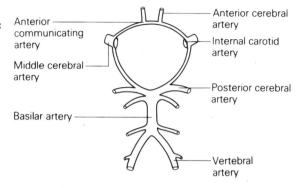

Effects of CVAs
Damage to **right** cerebral arteries leads to left-sided hemiplegia (paralysis) or hemiparesis (weakness)

Damage to **left** cerebral arteries leads to right-sided hemiplegia (paralysis) or hemiparesis (weakness)

Causes of cerebro-vascular accident
1   Cerebral thrombosis: a clot (thrombus) forms in a cerebral artery. Usually caused in the elderly by arteriosclerosis. Onset – gradual.
2   Cerebral haemorrhage: a cerebral artery ruptures caused by the pressure of hypertension. Onset – abrupt.
3   Cerebral embolism: a detached clot (embolus) lodges in one of the cerebral arteries, possibly following myocardial infarction. Onset – abrupt.

ADMISSION TO THE WARD

When Mrs Jones and her daughter arrive on the ward they are bewildered and apprehensive. They should both be made to feel welcome; a cup of tea makes any situation seem more normal.

The admitting nurse should explain the layout of the ward and introduce herself by name. Once Mrs Jones has settled into bed, a doctor will examine her and may speak to her daughter, but they will both want more information, particularly about the effects of the stroke. While admitting Mrs Jones, the nurse will have the opportunity to encourage and answer questions.

The doctor has decided that Mrs Jones has a left-sided hemiparesis, which means that there has been damage to her right cerebral arteries. Her left arm and leg have been affected by the stroke. If she had suffered damage to the left cerebral arteries, leading to right-sided hemiplegia or hemiparesis, she would probably also have suffered some effect on her speech (dysphasia).

<table>
<tr><td>NURSING CARE</td><td>

Initial stages

</td></tr>
</table>

NURSING CARE

Initial stages

It has been said that 'the nurse who handles the new hemiplegic patient on admission to hospital and in the very early days is the key member of any rehabilitation unit' (Johnstone, 1982). It is vital that all the nurses involved in Mrs Jones' care understand their role. Referral

Positioning a patient with left hemiplegia

Lying on the affected side   Lying on the unaffected side

Getting out of bed   Transferring to a chair

In order for rehabilitation to be realistic, an awareness of what Mrs Jones' home is like can be very helpful. Some Consultant Geriatricians arrange for photographs of the patient's home to be made available. More usually, an occupational therapist, occasionally accompanied by a ward nurse, goes with Mrs Jones to her home prior to the final discharge and advises on any modifications which might be helpful. For example, moving furniture or advising on aids which are available, particularly in the toilet, bathroom and kitchen.

Key members of the multidisciplinary team

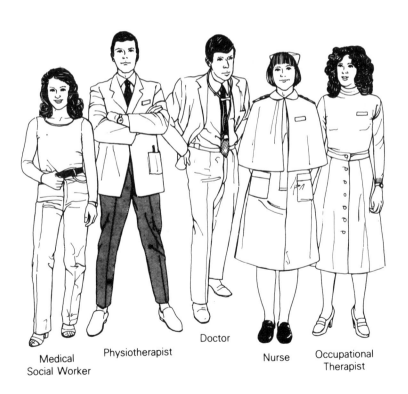

Medical
Social Worker

Physiotherapist

Doctor

Nurse

Occupational
Therapist

In order to ensure that the move from hospital to home is as smooth and troublefree as possible, the nurses on the ward complete a *discharge checklist*. This also helps to promote continuity of care from hospital ward into the community.

Discharge checklist

	Arranged by	Date	Remarks
Patient informed			
Relative informed			
Transport booked			
Home help			
Meals on Wheels			
Keys available			
Valuables from safe			
Day Hospital			
Day Centre			
Community nurse			
Letter to G.P.			
Drugs ordered			
Drugs on ward			
OPD appointment			
Part III place			
Warden informed			

COMMUNITY CARE

The medical social worker at the hospital has arranged with the Social Services Department that Mrs Jones will receive help with the housework twice a week by a home help. Meals on Wheels will be delivered three times a week. Her daughter has arranged to call in at weekends and twice a week Mrs Jones will be taken by ambulance to the Geriatric Day Hospital for follow-up rehabilitation.

The community liaison nurse from the hospital Geriatric Unit has arranged to call in and visit Mrs Jones one week following discharge to ensure that all is well. If she feels that home nursing care is required she will contact her colleague in the primary health care team to arrange it.

Mrs Jones has borrowed a tripod walking stick from the hospital and feels confident that with all the support made available to her, she will be able to continue living in her ground floor flat on her own.

TEST YOURSELF

Using this test as a guide, write notes on the following aspects of the preceding chapter. Ask your Tutor or Ward Sister to have a look at your notes to discuss any problems.

1 How would you describe the effects of a stroke to the wife of an elderly man who has suffered one? What advice would you give her as to how she can help in the rehabilitative process?

2 How many members of the multidisciplinary team have you met? How many more can you think of? What is the purpose of the case conference?

3 Do you think the use of a discharge checklist is a good idea? Make a list of all the problems that might occur when discharging an elderly person from hospital, then describe briefly how these problems could be prevented.

4   Cerebro-vascular accidents are more prevalent in people over the age of 65. Why do
you think this is the case?

FURTHER READING

CAIRD, F., KENNEDY, R. & WILLIAMS, B. 1983. *Practical Rehabilitation of the Elderly.* London: Pitman.

CONI, N., DAVISON, W. & WEBSTER, S. 1980. *Lecture Notes on Geriatrics*, 2nd ed. Oxford: Blackwell Scientific Publications.

JOHNSTONE, M. 1982. *The Stroke Patient: Principles of Rehabilitation*, 2nd ed. Edinburgh: Churchill Livingstone.

MYCO, F. 1983. *Nursing Care of the Hemiplegic Stroke Patient.* London: Harper and Row.

NORTON, D., MCLAREN, R., & EXTON-SMITH, A. 1962. *An Investigation of Geriatric Nursing Problems in Hospital.* National Corporation for the Care of Old People. (Reprinted 1976, Churchill Livingstone.)

WORLD HEALTH ORGANIZATION. 1971. 'Stroke–Treatment, Rehabilitation and Prevention,' *WHO Chronicle*, 25 Oct.

4 Mr Arkwright who is admitted to the ward with chronic bronchitis/emphysema

HISTORY

Mr Arkwright is a 72 year old retired road-sweeper who lives with his wife in a first floor flat in the middle of a busy city centre. He has always been a heavy smoker, suffering with a smoker's cough for most of his adult life.

He has had several spells in hospital with bronchitis. Despite repeated advice from nursing and medical staff he has not given up smoking. During one mild and damp November, Mr Arkwright has a particularly severe attack of breathlessness while negotiating the stairs to the flat.

His wife calls their G.P. who arranges with the local hospital that Mr Arkwright should be admitted to the Geriatric Unit. The G.P. books an ambulance and Mrs Arkwright packs a suitcase and accompanies her husband to the hospital.

Predisposing factors to bronchitis:

smoking
polluted environment
(fog, smoke, etc.)
dusty work

ADMISSION TO HOSPITAL

The nurses on the ward of the Geriatric Unit are awaiting Mr Arkwright's arrival and a bed with a sheepskin underblanket to protect his pressure areas has been prepared in a warm, well-ventilated corner of the ward.

Mrs Arkwright helps him to undress and put his pyjamas on and with the aid of a nurse he gets into bed. As he is very breathless, the

33

nurse ensures that he is sitting upright, well-supported with pillows. She finds that Mr and Mrs Arkwright understand the illness fairly well but recognise that on this occasion he seems more ill than ever before.

DIAGNOSIS

Following medical examination, the doctor diagnoses *acute exacerbation of chronic bronchitis with emphysema*. While the admitting nurse takes a nursing history in order to identify nursing problems and plan care, Mr and Mrs Arkwright are able to ask her to explain the diagnosis.

The lungs

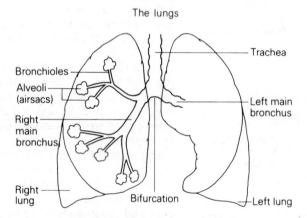

RESPIRATORY INFECTION
AND/OR PREDISPOSING FACTORS
↓
ACUTE BRONCHITIS
inflammation of bronchi, oversecretion of mucus, wheeze, cough, sputum, dypsnoea
↓
CHRONIC BRONCHITIS
chronic inflammation of the bronchi, recurrent infective exacerbations, hypersecretion of mucus, dypsnoea, cough, purulent copious sputum
↓
EMPHYSEMA

Emphysema
distension of the alveoli (airsacs) of the lungs
characterised by 'barrel' chest, dypsnoea and cyanosis,
persistent cough, scant sputum.

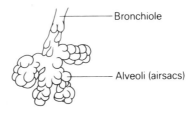

Bronchiole

Alveoli (airsacs)

1 chronic bronchitis causes increasing obstruction of
   bronchi and bronchioles with mucus
2 inspired air cannot escape through narrowed bronchi
   and bronchioles
3 airsacs (alveoli) become increasingly distended with
   air
4 thin walls of alveoli break down
5 capillary networks surrounding alveoli break down
6 which eventually causes cardiac failure

MEDICAL TREATMENT

Medical treatment:

broad spectrum
antibiotic

intermittent
oxygen

bronchodilator

expectorant

physiotherapy
(chest percussion
and postural
drainage)

Although there is no cure for chronic bronchitis and emphysema, the acute infective exacerbation can be treated and the symptoms relieved.

The doctor stresses that it would help Mr Arkwright enormously in relieving some of his symptoms if he could stop smoking. Mrs Arkwright undertakes to throw away all his cigarettes and he agrees to try and give up once again.

NURSING CARE

Initial stages

The nursing staff notice that Mr Arkwright is particularly agitated when his wife goes home, and that she seems unusually depressed. He sleeps very badly during his first night despite

35

the fact that his breathlessness is less severe and he assures the nurses that he is comfortable.

The following day when his wife visits, one of the nurses who admitted him spends time talking to the couple and discovers that he has never been a patient on a Geriatric Ward before. Both Mr Arkwright and his wife are convinced that he will never go home again.

Fortunately the nurse is able to allay their fears, and explain that geriatric care does not necessarily mean longstay care.

Initially Mr Arkwright is nursed in an upright position in bed and encouraged to move himself about regularly to ease his pressure points. He is encouraged to drink plenty of fluids and manages to eat a light, easily digested, attractively presented diet.

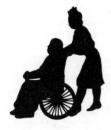

He is constipated on admission and requires a laxative, following which he asks for a bran-based cereal for breakfast every morning. He finds using the commode an embarrassing impossibility, preferring to be taken to the toilet in a wheelchair until he is able to walk there himself.

PHYSIOTHERAPY

The physiotherapist becomes an important part of his life, combining chest percussion with postural drainage and teaching him breathing exercises. As the acute phase of his illness subsides, she encourages him to become more mobile gradually. Everyone involved in his care is delighted to see his efforts to give up smoking.

Some facts about smoking:

1 Smoking leads to more deaths from heart attacks than it does to deaths from any other disease
2 Cigarette smoking is a very important cause of diseases of the leg arteries

3 Women who smoke when they are pregnant run a greater risk of miscarriage or of their baby being born premature or underweight
4 Among 1000 young men who smoke, about 6 will be killed on the roads but about 250 will be killed before their time by tobacco

Source: The Health Education Council

Planning discharge

Mr Arkwright's condition slowly improves and he is able to move around the ward at his own pace, stopping for frequent rests to 'catch his breath'. He dislikes sitting in the dayroom with the other patients. His attempts to give up smoking make him irritable and unable to concentrate on cardgames or reading or television.

The occupational therapist assesses his ability to dress himself and the nursing staff encourage Mrs Arkwright to visit in the morning to help him get out of bed, wash and dress. She is advised on the best methods of helping without doing too much and without harming herself.

A date is finally agreed for Mr Arkwright's discharge and the medical social worker sees the couple together to ensure that they will be able to cope. As Mr Arkwright will be attending the Day Hospital once a week, Mrs Arkwright feels that there is a lifeline of support.

Mr Arkwright visits the Day Hospital prior to his discharge and the physiotherapist there assesses his capability to climb stairs. With frequent halts, he is able to manage and the arrangements for his discharge go ahead.

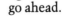

37

DISCHARGE

Mr Arkwright's discharge is uneventful. An ambulance collects him in the morning to take him home and the ambulance crew helps him to manoeuvre the stairs. Despite the fact that he has been spending every day out of bed, dressed and walking around in the hospital ward, his wife has prepared for him to go to bed as soon as he gets home as she thinks he will be tired.

However, he settles into a comfortable armchair in front of the fire with a cup of tea. When the Geriatric Liaison Nurse visits him the following day to check that all is well and that he understands the arrangements regarding the Day Hospital, she finds that he has already started smoking again.

VISITING THE DAY HOSPITAL

Mr and Mrs Arkwright know that an ambulance will collect him in the morning on the day of his visit to the Day Hospital and also bring him back again.

So that the ambulance crew does not have to wait, Mr Arkwright is up and dressed with his hat and coat on by half past eight. The ambulance arrives to collect him at ten o'clock, having collected several other day patients from the district first.

They arrive at the Day Hospital about half an hour later having collected another patient. A nurse takes Mr Arkwright's hat and coat, gives him coffee and shows him to a seat with some other patients.

Eventually he is seen by a doctor whom he has never met before and is given a thorough medical examination. The doctor seems reasonably satisfied with him and a nurse escorts him back into the main body of the

Reasons for attending Day Hospital:

medical treatment, assessment or follow-up

rehabilitative maintenance

nursing treatment

chiropody

respite for carers

Day Hospital, a large room with smaller rooms leading off. He is pleased to see that the toilets are clearly marked.

After lunch a nurse helps Mr Arkwright to have a bath and explains something of the routine of the Day Hospital. He is to be seen by the physiotherapist after his bath, then it will be time for tea and home.

As the weeks progress Mr Arkwright finds that the people attending Day Hospital on 'his' day have a wide variety of different ailments and are all there for different reasons. He knows that his wife appreciates the few free hours to shop and clean and visit friends without having to worry about him.

He is seen regularly by the doctor and it is the decision of the team during a discussion about Mr Arkwright that it will be to his own benefit and his wife's if he continues to attend Day Hospital once a week.

On one day a week, at least, his cigarette smoking will be curtailed.

Some facts about Day Hospitals:

a day hospital of 40 day places caters for up to 200 elderly people a week

Diagnoses in 222 patients attending day hospital

Stroke	86	Respiratory disease	7
Arthritis	51	Depression	8
Parkinsonism	11	Leg ulcer	6
Amputation	10	Femoral fracture	2
Paraplegia	9	Incontinence	2
Dementia	9	Other	21

Source: Brocklehurst and Tucker (1982)

TEST YOURSELF	Do you think you can answer the following questions after reading this chapter? You may need to refer to other books or talk to your Tutor or Ward Sister.

1 What are the risk factors associated with smoking? Do you think the team was right to try and stop the patient from smoking?

Do you know how to obtain literature from your local Health Education Council about smoking? How can nurses influence the smoking habits of patients?

2 Describe the function of the Day Hospital. What is the difference between a Day Hospital and a Day Centre? Where is the nearest Day Centre to your hospital? Could you arrange a visit to it through your Tutor?

3 What is meant by 'postural drainage'? How could you find out about the practical aspects of this form of therapy?

4 If a patient was admitted to the geriatric ward on which you were working, what would you say and do to reassure him or her?

FURTHER READING

BARROWCLOUGH, F. & PINEL, C. 1979. *Geriatric Care for Nurses*. London: Heinemann Medical.

BROCKLEHURST, J. & TUCKER, J. 1982. *Progress in Geriatric Day Care*. King Edward's Hospital Fund. Oxford: Oxford University Press.

FERGUSON ANDERSON, W., CAIRD, F., KENNEDY, R. & SCHWARTZ, D. 1982. *Gerontology and Geriatric Nursing*. Sevenoaks: Hodder and Stoughton.

GREEN, J. 1979. *Basic Clinical Physiology*. Oxford: Oxford University Press.

5 Mrs Booth who is admitted to the ward with diabetes mellitus

Mrs Booth is a 74 year old lady living in a seaside resort on the South Coast. At the beginning of her 60s she was diagnosed as suffering from *diabetes mellitus* which has been controlled with tablets and with a reducing diet as she is overweight.

What is diabetes mellitus?
A disorder of carbohydrate metabolism due to failure of the pancreas to produce insulin causing the blood glucose to be persistently raised above the normal range.

Special features about mature-onset diabetes:

Often detected accidentally, during routine urinalysis

Occurs most commonly between 65–74
Glucose tolerance declines with age
Risk of complications greater

A permanent slight hyperglycaemia is desirable due to the dangerous effects of hypoglycaemic attacks

Mature-onset diabetes mellitus

signs and symptoms

thirst/polydipsia/dryness of mouth/glycosuria/pruritis vulvae/balanitis/polyuria/frequency of urine

Mrs Booth's husband has recently died and a few weeks following her bereavement a Health Visitor calls to see how she is coping, knowing that she has no close relatives or friends. Her husband was the focal point of her life and so the Health Visitor knows that Mrs Booth will be missing him very much indeed.

In fact, she finds that Mrs Booth seems withdrawn and rather muddled and her speech is

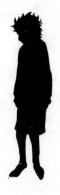

slurred. She looks generally unkempt and appears not to be eating regular meals. It does seem, however, that she has automatically been taking the medication prescribed to control her diabetes.

The Health Visitor suspects that Mrs Booth's mental confusion is due to *hypoglycaemia* caused by her failure to eat regularly while continuing her medication. She manages to persuade Mrs Booth to have a cup of tea sweetened with two heaped teaspoons of sugar.

Hypoglycaemia
Deficiency of sugar in the blood

Hypoglycaemic attacks in the elderly characterised by:

mental confusion/behaviour disorders
slurred speech
sleep disturbance
rapid pulse
sweatiness

and can lead to:

permanent neurological damage
if uncorrected

In view of Mrs Booth's general debility, the Health Visitor decides to recommend to her G.P. that a short period in hospital will be of benefit. Mrs Booth is too apathetic to be particularly concerned. An ambulance is arranged and she is taken to the admission ward of the Geriatric Unit of the local hospital.

ADMISSION TO HOSPITAL

Fortunately, Mrs Booth arrives on the admission ward at a particularly tranquil period of the day – the late afternoon. The admitting nurse is able to spend some time talking to her, showing her the ward and helping her to unpack her case, hastily packed by the Health Visitor.

Mrs Booth, however, remains withdrawn and appears disorientated. She refuses a cup of tea and is disinterested in the attempts of the nurse to explain the layout of the ward.

A doctor examines her soon after her arrival on the ward and identifies physical problems related to her diabetes. He finds that she is suffering from peripheral vascular disease and has a small superficial ischaemic ulcer on her left foot.

Complications of mature-onset diabetes mellitus:

cataract: diabetic retinopathy
sensory neuropathy, especially of the legs
renal damage: albuminuria
arteriosclerosis
peripheral vascular disease
susceptibility to infection

NURSING CARE

Initial stages

Mrs Booth refuses supper but accepts a hot milky drink and some biscuits. The nurse who admitted her notices that she remains withdrawn and monosyllabic and that she is obviously tired following the disruption caused by her admission to hospital. All she wants to do is go to bed.

Deciding that there is little to be gained in trying to persuade Mrs Booth to have a much-needed bath or wash that evening, the nurse helps her into bed having first managed to obtain a specimen of urine.

A bed cradle is placed in the bed to keep the weight of the covers off Mrs Booth's legs and feet and a sheepskin underblanket helps to protect her pressure areas. The nurse notices that the ischaemic ulcer on Mrs Booth's left foot appears to be healing but that a visit from the chiropodist will be needed.

Ischaemia of the lower limbs:

Arteriosclerosis affects blood supply to lower limbs ie abdominal aorta,
iliac, femoral, popliteal arteries

Signs and symptoms
pain in calf during exercise
intermittent claudication, relieved by resting

rest pain in feet due to severe arterial insufficiency may lead to painful superficial ulcers and possibly to gangrene of toes/heel, sepsis and even amputation

ischaemic lesions are most common in older male patients

NURSING CARE

Rehabilitation

Several members of the multidisciplinary team are closely involved in Mrs Booth's rehabilitation. On her first morning in the ward after a good night's sleep the night nursing staff note that she is not at all confused, although still apparently withdrawn.

After breakfast and a bath, she is gently persuaded to dress in her own clothes and join some of the other patients in the day room.

Mrs Booth is interviewed by the dietitian who tries to ascertain her likes and dislikes in relation to food so that a realistic diet can be made up for her. Mrs Booth's dietary habits were already well-established before she was diagnosed as suffering from diabetes. Some compromises in her diet have already been made in the past few years. Nevertheless, a sensible diet which will prevent weight gain and excessive hyperglycaemia is important.

Her medication is continued as before and daily urinalysis following the main meal of the day is undertaken by the nursing staff.

Mrs Booth is also seen by the chiropodist whose particular skills are needed to ensure that no trauma occurs to her skin when her

Better Cookery for Diabetics
An illustrated cookery book prepared by Jill Metcalfe, a dietitian of the British Diabetic Association, containing practical hints for following the low fat, high fibre diet recommended for diabetics.

toenails are cut. Her poor peripheral circulation means that any lesion to her extremities will heal very slowly. She will also be more prone to developing infection in any areas of broken skin as a result of her diabetes.

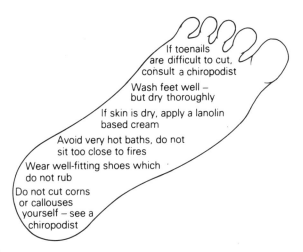

If toenails are difficult to cut, consult a chiropodist

Wash feet well – but dry thoroughly

If skin is dry, apply a lanolin based cream

Avoid very hot baths, do not sit too close to fires

Wear well-fitting shoes which do not rub

Do not cut corns or callouses yourself – see a chiropodist

After a period of two weeks on the geriatric assessment ward, Mrs Booth's physical condition gradually improves; she is now able to walk without help, wash and dress herself, and an appointment has been booked to assess her cooking skills in the kitchen of the Occupational Therapy Department.

Despite her physical improvement, the team note that Mrs Booth remains rather withdrawn. She is disinterested in ward activities and no one has been able to persuade her to discuss the reason for the breakdown in her physical health.

However, as discussions about her discharge home gather momentum, the medical social worker is able to take her into a quiet, private corner of the ward to discuss her finances and whether she needs any help.

For the first time since her admission, Mrs Booth begins to talk unreservedly. It is obvious that she is still devastated by the death of her husband. The couple had been lively and popular but Mrs Booth has found her circle of friends diminishing since his death.

Missing him desperately, she finds her friends embarrassed when she talks about him. Consequently she has felt increasingly isolated and found it difficult to cope managing the bungalow.

Planning discharge

Having discussed Mrs Booth's progress, the multidisciplinary team is satisfied that her physical condition is stable. The small ischaemic ulcer on her foot has almost healed and her diabetes is controlled.

However, there is concern over how she can best be supported emotionally. Her reaction to the death of her husband is absolutely normal and the prescribing of antidepressants or tranquillisers would be inappropriate and of no value.

A plan of action offering a range of statutory services is suggested to Mrs Booth, together with suggestions as to where else she can turn to for help if she wishes:

financial advice from the medical social worker
weekly monitoring visit to Day Hospital
Age Concern Luncheon Club
contact with 'Cruse'
immediate follow-up visit by community liaison nurse
referral to Health Visitor
?referral to Community Psychiatric Nurse

What have you learnt from this chapter? Test yourself with these questions and refer to your Tutor or Ward Sister for advice on anything still puzzling you.

1 Have you ever met a Community Psychiatric Nurse? Are there any Community Psychiatric Nurses in your area who specialise in the care of the elderly? What is their function and how can you contact them?

2 Imagine you are an elderly diabetic. Plan your menu for a week after working out what your income is likely to be. How can you find out about financial benefits? Have you ever visited a Luncheon Club?

3 Do you know what a 'death grant' is? When a patient on your ward dies, what immediate practical advice can you offer about the procedures for dealing with a death – registering the death, collecting the death certificate, and so on.

4 How would you recognise a hypoglycaemic attack in a diabetic patient? How would you deal with it?

FURTHER READING

BRITISH DIABETIC ASSOCIATION. 1970. *The Care of the Elderly Diabetic.*
BRITISH DIABETIC ASSOCIATION. 1980. *Care of the Feet*, Leaflet DH107.
OAKLEY, W. G., PYKE, D. A. & TAYLOR, K. W. 1978. *Diabetes and its Management*, 3rd ed. Oxford: Blackwell Scientific Publications.
PITT, B. 1982. *Psychogeriatrics: An Introduction to the Psychiatry of Old Age.* Edinburgh: Churchill Livingstone.

6

Mrs Tybalt who is admitted to the ward with arthritis and is overweight

HISTORY

Association of Carers:

Profile of membership – April 1983

Sex of carer
female	79.78%
male	20.22%

Age of carer
20–29	1.38%
30–39	9.63%
40–49	15.13%
50–59	35.08%
60–69	28.20%
70+	10.59%

Sex of dependant
female	55.68%
male	39.74%
child	6.58%

Mrs Tybalt has lived with her only daughter and son-in-law in a pleasant suburban house for five years since the death of her husband. She is 82 and her daughter is 53, with three children who are all married and have left home.

Mrs Tybalt suffers with osteoarthritis and is very overweight, weighing about 12 stone. She has her own room on the ground floor of the house with a commode. Her osteoarthritic knee joints have made negotiating the stairs to the toilet a virtual impossibility.

Mrs Tybalt needs help from her daughter to wash, dress and get out of bed. She spends most of her days reading and snoozing and is very fond of a cup of tea and a biscuit or a piece of cake. She has become increasingly immobile as the pain in her knees has discouraged her from walking.

Mrs Tybalt's daughter Janet gave up her job as a teacher to look after her mother. Her husband travels away from home a good deal as part of his work and Janet is beginning to feel the strain as her mother becomes increasingly forgetful and demanding as well as physically exhausting.

DOMICILIARY VISIT

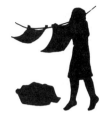

Recently Mrs Tybalt has suffered several incidents of urinary incontinence, involving a tremendous amount of additional laundering of bedlinen and clothing for Janet. Finally, following an episode of faecal incontinence after several days of constipation, Janet calls in the G.P. pleading that her mother be admitted to hospital to give her a rest.

The doctor recognises that Janet is under considerable stress and contacts the Geriatric Unit of the local hospital to request that a Consultant Geriatrician from the hospital make a domiciliary visit. Accompanied by the Department's Community Liaison Nurse, the Geriatrician visits the Tybalts at home at the earliest opportunity.

Domiciliary visit

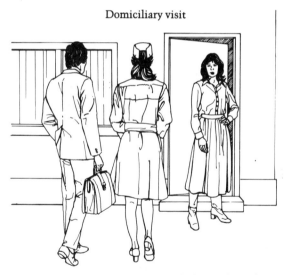

Having examined Mrs Tybalt and spoken privately to her daughter, the Geriatrician and nurse decide that the whole family will benefit if Mrs Tybalt is admitted to the Geriatric Unit for a period of assessment and rehabilitation.

ADMISSION TO HOSPITAL

Somewhat apprehensive and upset at having her comfortable, established routine thrown into turmoil, Mrs Tybalt is accompanied to the hospital by her daughter late the following afternoon. Janet is beginning to regret her impetuousness in calling the doctor in the first place and is a little alarmed by the unexpectedly clinical atmosphere of the geriatic admission ward.

Recognising the apprehension of mother and daughter, the admitting nurse takes time to explain the mysteries of the ward. Janet is relieved to discover that she will be free to visit at any time. Having already spoken to the community liaison nurse, the nurse on the ward stresses the expected temporary nature of the admission. Having helped her mother to settle into bed, Janet unpacks her mother's clothes and goes home.

A doctor examines Mrs Tybalt, diagnosing her as suffering from *osteoarthrosis, obesity,* with a suspected *urinary tract infection* and *faecal impaction.*

Osteoarthrosis
(Degenerative joint disease)

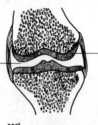

degeneration of articular cartilage, reduction of joint space, sclerosis of bone, formation of 'spurs'

Synovial membrane — Articular cartilage

A very large number of elderly people may show radiological evidence of osteoarthritic joint degeneration. Mainly asymptomatic	Predisposing factors are obesity and previous trauma. Exact causes unknown	Where symptoms occur, they include pain, stiffness, swelling, deformity (e.g. Heberden's nodules of terminal finger joints)	Osteoarthritic changes most commonly occur in hands and lower limbs

Initial stages

In planning nursing care, the priorities of Mrs Tybalt's needs are quickly established. The immediate concern is to solve the demoralising problem of her faecal incontinence. She appears to be suffering with diarrhoea, but the leakage of liquid faeces is in fact due to *impaction of faeces*. The doctor suspects that constipation has been caused by the codeine compound she has been taking for the pain due to her osteoarthrosis.

Faecal impaction:

constipation leading to accumulation of mass of faeces in rectum leading to oozing of liquid faeces around impaction

Immediate treatment
Mild cases: suppositories
Worse cases: enemata
Severe cases: manual (digital) evacuation

Follow-up treatment: prevention
Privacy and plenty of time to go to the toilet
Roughage in diet, bran-based breakfast cereal
Laxatives and aperients if necessary

With some difficulty, a specimen of urine is finally obtained from Mrs Tybalt to exclude infection as a cause of her urinary incontinence which has only started relatively recently.

Plan of action:

Pain control
Reducing diet
Physiotherapy
Occupational
therapy

In the event, she is found not to have a urinary tract infection and the team feels that her urinary incontinence may be caused by her unwillingness to cause pain in her joints when moving in and out of chair or bed to get to the toilet or commode.

Rehabilitation

Mrs Tybalt's daughter is very anxious about her mother's hospitalisation. Accustomed to doing virtually everything for her mother and to giving her frequent sweet 'treats', she is alarmed at the energetic programme of rehabilitation which her mother seems to be subjected to.

Present on the ward for most of the day, Janet finds her mother's diet frugal; the sweet 'treats' have been very firmly banned.

To eat

lean meats
fresh fruit
fresh vegetables
low calorie soft drinks
skimmed milk
low fat cheeses

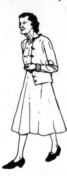

And not to eat

sweets
cakes
jams
sugar
milk
cheese

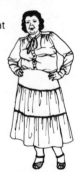

The team involved in Mrs Tybalt's care realises at a very early stage that Janet is not happy about her mother's treatment and begin to involve her more and more in the rehabilitation programme. Mrs Tybalt, whose morale has improved considerably with the curing of her faecal incontinence, becomes less irritable with her daughter as Janet becomes more constructively involved rather than simply worrying and fussing.

Janet is encouraged to accompany her mother to the Physiotherapy and Occupational Therapy Departments and is surprised at how much her mother is able to do for herself. She is made aware of the benefits to them both if Mrs Tybalt is able to lose more weight and gain more independence.

Mrs Tybalt, spoiled by her daughter since the death of her husband and discouraged from doing anything to help in the house because Janet found it quicker and easier to do it herself, is beginning to take on a new lease of life.

**Drugs commonly
used for
musculo-skeletal
pain relief:**

paracetamol
distalgesic
aspirin
codeine
ibuprofen
indomethacin
pentazocine
phenylbutazone

Planning discharge

The multidisciplinary team is aware that osteoarthrosis is a degenerative disease which cannot be reversed. While surgical intervention in the form of joint replacement is certainly an acceptable mode of treatment where sufferers are subjected to severe pain, in Mrs Tybalt's case this is not felt to be appropriate. Her pain is now well under control with medication prescribed by the doctor.

Following discussions between members of the team, it is decided that an occupational therapist will accompany Mrs Tybalt home for an afternoon visit to ascertain whether any aids might be usefully provided. Mrs Tybalt and the occupational therapist accompanied by a nurse are ferried to Mrs Tybalt's home by ambulance to be greeted by Janet.

The family has been coping with Mrs Tybalt in her ground floor room for many years and discovered for themselves a variety of ways to make life easier. The bed is fairly high, the armchair has a springlift seat and there is a commode in the room.

The occupational therapist is able to suggest a variety of other aids which will help Mrs Tybalt to retain some independence: Velcro clothes fastenings, slip-on shoes or elastic shoe laces, stocking aids, a raised toilet seat.

DISCHARGE

The trial home visit has helped in many ways; Mrs Tybalt's daughter is grateful to have had the opportunity to discuss her mother's disabilities with both a nurse and an occupational therapist, feeling that they now understand her situation properly having been to see it for themselves.

The hospital staff in their turn have been

Discharge plan:

day hospital once weekly
supply of analgesics
reducing diet sheet
follow-up visit by community liaison nurse
'respite bed' every year

able to assess Mrs Tybalt's capabilities realistically, and Mrs Tybalt herself finally knows beyond doubt that she will eventually be going home again for good. The date for discharge is agreed for one week following the home visit.

'RESPITE' CARE

The Tybalts are fortunate to be living in an area where it is established practice to set aside beds within the Geriatric Unit where elderly dependants can be admitted for one to two week periods. This enables their carers to have a short break, even a holiday, which would otherwise be impossible.

Coupled with the weekly Day Hospital visit and follow-up care from the Primary Health Care Team, Mrs Tybalt's daughter feels that she can cope a little more optimistically.

The visiting Health Visitor ensures that Janet is aware of several supportive charitable organisations which might be of help – the Association of Carers, the National Council for Carers and Their Dependants, and the Arthritis and Rheumatism Council.

Janet no longer feels quite so isolated.

TEST YOURSELF

See if you can answer the following questions – ask your Tutor or Ward Sister for help if there are some you have difficulty with.

1   Do you know the common causes of constipation in the elderly? What would lead you to suspect that a patient was suffering with faecal impaction? How would you treat it? Describe in detail the design and proper use of an incontinence bedpad.

2   What is the role of a continence adviser? What are the advantages of the post to

other nurses? Do you think there is a need for this type of specialist nurse?

3 What is the purpose of a domiciliary visit? Do nurses accompany doctors on domiciliary visits from your hospital? Why?

4 Many elderly people are cared for at home by relatives or friends. Describe some of the difficulties that the carer might experience. What statutory services are available in your area to help support carers?

FURTHER READING

Action on Incontinence – Report of a Working Group. 1983. London: King's Fund Project Paper.

ARTHRITIS AND RHEUMATISM COUNCIL. *A Handbook for Patients: Osteoarthritis (Osteoarthrosis).*

CAIRD, F. & JUDGE, T. 1982. *Drug Treatment of the Elderly Patient.* London: Pitman Medical.

EASTMAN, M. 1984. *Old Age Abuse.* Age Concern (England).

FAMILY POLICY STUDIES CENTRE. 1984. *The Forgotten Army: Family Care and Elderly People.* London: Family Policy Studies Centre.

HUGHES, S. 1983. *Aston's Short Textbook of Orthopaedics and Traumatology,* 3rd ed. Sevenoaks: Hodder and Stoughton.

ROYAL COLLEGE OF NURSING. 1982. *The Problems of Promoting Continence.* London: Royal College of Nursing.

WILLINGTON, F. L. 1976. *Incontinence in the Elderly.* London: Academic Press.

7 Miss Perrin who is admitted to the ward suffering from hypothermia

HISTORY

Miss Perrin, 85, lives alone in a large terraced house in the suburbs of a busy industrial city. Since the death of her sister with whom she had shared her home for many years she has become rather reclusive. She relies on a neighbour to do her weekly shopping and collect her pension.

One wintry evening in January the neighbour calls on her weekly visit but is unable to get any reply. Very concerned, she calls the police who are able to find a way into the house.

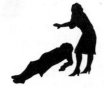

The police find Miss Perrin lying on the floor in her nightdress outside her bedroom. She seems confused and disorientated and is very cold to touch. The police wrap her in a blanket and call for an ambulance to take her to the Accident and Emergency Department at the local hospital.

Clinical examination at the hospital reveals that Miss Perrin has a rectal temperature of 33°C. She is admitted to the geriatric assessment ward with a diagnosis of *accidental hypothermia*.

Accidental hypothermia:
(body core temperature falls below 35°C)

Predisposing factors

Immobility	Living alone	Confusion
Falls	Depression	Dementia

Cold environment: poor housing, poor heating, cold
weather

Poor nutritional status   Myxoedema
Some drugs: phenothiazines, barbiturates
Excessive alcohol intake
Ineffective thermo-regulation

Clinical features
Cold skin, especially abdomen and groins
Puffy, pinkish skin
Rectal temperature below 35°C
Progressive slowing of pulse
Progressive fall of blood pressure
Slow shallow respirations
Lethargy and sluggishness
Progressive confusion and disorientation
BELOW 32°C = Muscular rigidity
                              Unconsciousness
                              Death

ADMISSION TO THE WARD

Miss Perrin is still very drowsy and confused on arrival at the geriatric admission ward. She is put to bed in a warm sideroom where the temperature is about 23°C. A large cell ripple mattress has been placed on the bed to help protect her pressure areas.

The nurses are aware that if Miss Perrin's temperature rises too quickly, peripheral vasodilation could lead to a fatal drop in blood pressure. She is wrapped in a heat-retaining metallised blanket but excessive extra blankets are not loaded on to the bed and hot water bottles are strictly forbidden.

Medical treatment:

oxygen therapy as
necessary
broad spectrum
antibiotic
fluid replacement
IV hydrocortisone

The admitting doctor examines Miss Perrin briefly, unwilling to expose her unnecessarily. He orders the relevant treatment with the intention of assessing her again the following day.

Initial stages

Miss Perrin's temperature is checked rectally with a lowgrade thermometer every hour with the aim that there should be a rise of about 0.6°C hourly. This is a difficult procedure for the nursing staff as Miss Perrin remains confused and somewhat restless.

While one nurse checks the position and reading of the thermometer, the other talks gently to Miss Perrin, explaining repetitively where she is and what is happening. During this contact with their patient, the nurses notice that Miss Perrin seems to be covered in bruises not concomitant with her recent incident. They record this observation in the nursing notes.

Hypothermia: initial nursing care

Check rectal temperature hourly with lowgrade thermometer
Check pulse, respirations, and blood pressure hourly
Give warm fluids if patient is conscious
Nurse patient in warm room (23°C)
Protect pressure areas
Maintain patient's hygiene
Give high carbohydrate foods if possible

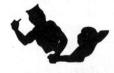

On the morning following Miss Perrin's admission to hospital, her temperature has stabilised at 36.5°C and she appears to have recovered both mentally and physically. She is able to sit out in an armchair with help after having had a wash and she enjoys a nourishing breakfast.

Examining her more fully than when she was admitted, the doctor is able to ascertain exactly what had caused the incidence of hypothermia. During an early morning visit to the toilet, Miss Perrin had fallen heavily and was unable to get to her feet again as she felt very faint and giddy. For nearly eight hours she had been lying on the floor.

PHYSICAL INSTABILITY

The doctor's attention had already been drawn to the bruises on Miss Perrin's arms and legs by the nursing staff. Gentle quizzing reveals that she has become increasingly prone to falling down, especially in the morning when getting out of bed.

Some common causes of falls in the elderly

Environmental
Poor lighting
Slippery floors
Loose floor coverings
Trailing flexes
Stairs
Obstacles
Ill-fitting footwear
Pets

Physical
Postural hypotension
Transient ischaemic attacks
Epilepsy
Parkinsonism
Peripheral neuropathy
Drugs
'Drop' attacks
Failing sight
Cervical spondylosis

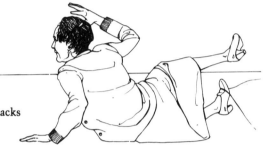

The doctor establishes that following the death of her sister, Miss Perrin had been prescribed a sedative by her G.P. and had been receiving repeat prescriptions for the same sedative drug ever since. He suspects that she is suffering from *postural hypotension* as a result of the effects of the drug.

Postural hypotension:

prolonged fall in blood pressure on standing up from a sitting or lying position

causes
some drugs, e.g. hypotensive agents, diuretics, sedatives, vasodilators

diseases of the autonomic nervous system

Rehabilitation

As Miss Perrin recovers from the physical effects of her accident, she is encouraged to become more independent. Her neighbour has visited and brought clothes and personal belongings so Miss Perrin is able to dress in her own clothes, wearing well-fitting, comfortable shoes. She is advised on how to try and overcome the effects of postural hypotension.

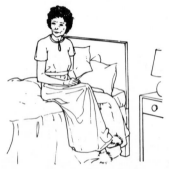

Overcoming postural hypotension:

take your time getting up in the morning
sit on the edge of the bed for a while
sit on the edge of the bed to get dressed
never stand up suddenly
always take your time
wear elastic stockings

Pressure sores:

predisposing factors to development
friction and shearing

circulatory disorders

bony protuberances

incontinence

immobility

drug therapy, e.g. sedation

malnutrition and dietary deficiencies

anaemia

Miss Perrin has lost a good deal of confidence because of her falls and is very nervous about walking without someone beside her. The occupational therapist and physiotherapist are better able to grade her exercises knowing her diagnosis. Initially she uses a Zimmer frame but as her confidence increases she is able to walk using only a stick.

Miss Perrin, a retired teacher, is a very correct and reserved lady who has not been particularly forthcoming in talking about herself. As her rehabilitation programme has progressed, she has required less and less nursing help.

However, one day when about to be helped to have a bath by a member of the nursing staff, she volunteers the information that she has a very sore area on her hip. On investigation, it transpires that she has developed a pressure sore, almost certainly as a result of the length of time she lay on the floor prior to admission.

Fortunately, the nurses find that the level of damage to Miss Perrin's skin is slight. There is a small area of broken skin but the damage is superficial. Although the area around the sore is very red, it appears that the skin is granulating.

The nurses advise Miss Perrin to keep the area dry and not to put any unnecessary pressure on the affected hip – in other words, not to lie on it in bed.

NURSING CARE

Planning discharge

As plans for her discharge are discussed, Miss Perrin confesses to the medical social worker during a private discussion that with her increasing age she does not relish the prospect of staying on her own in the large, lonely terraced house.

The house is difficult to maintain and heat, and is inconvenient as she grows less nimble. She is particularly afraid of a repeat of the incident which has led to this episode of hypothermia.

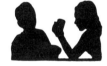

Various options are discussed with Miss Perrin as to where else she might be housed. Eventually she decides that with her small amount of savings plus the proceeds she could get from the sale of her house, she can afford to move into a private home.

The medical social worker advises her that a private nursing home rather than a Residential Care Home will probably suit her needs best and stresses that she should make all the arrangements at her own pace.

Miss Perrin's solicitor is an old family friend and following her discharge from hospital, with the help of her neighbour, arrangements are made for her to sell her house and move into a private nursing home.

Can you answer the following questions? Some of the answers are to be found in this chapter, some you will have to find out for yourself – perhaps your Tutor or Ward Sister can help.

1   How would you recognise a patient with hypothermia? Why is it dangerous to raise the temperature of a hypothermic patient quickly? What advice could you give to an old person living alone to guard against hypothermia?

2   What is the difference between a private residential care home and a private nursing home? What statutory control is there over private homes? If a patient wanted advice on selling property and entering private care, who would you advise them to go to?

3   What is postural hypotension? What advice would you give a patient with postural hypotension to help prevent falls?

4   What does 'iatrogenic disease' mean? Discuss the implications of iatrogenic disease in relation to the care of the elderly.

FURTHER READING

CENTRE FOR POLICY ON AGEING. 1984. *A Code of Practice for Residential Care Homes.* Folkestone, Kent: Bailey Brothers and Swinfen Ltd.

GOLDBERG, E. M. & CONNELLY, N. 1982. *The Effectiveness of Social Care for the Elderly.* London: Heinemann Educational.

TINKER, A. Department of the Environment. 1984. *Staying at Home: Helping Elderly People.* London: Her Majesty's Stationery Office.

WICKS, M. 1978. *Old and Cold: Hypothermia and Social Policy.* London: Heinemann Educational.

8 Continuing care

HISTORY

Two years ago Queenie Bloomington slipped on the icy pathway of her back garden on her way to the outside lavatory of her tiny terraced house. She fractured the neck of her femur and required insertion of a prosthesis hip replacement. Medical investigations showed her to be suffering from *osteoporosis*.

Osteoporosis:

development of a porous structure in bone

Very common disorder of old age, usually without symptoms but can cause back pain due to vertebral collapse, and predisposes to fractures.

Following the operation, Queenie suffered several setbacks. She developed a chest infection and a urinary tract infection and her wound was very slow to heal. This in turn affected her attempts at walking and after a stay of several months in the orthopaedic ward, she was referred to a Consultant Geriatrician. The Geriatrician visited Queenie and decided that she should be transferred to a geriatric rehabilitation ward.

NURSING CARE

Rehabilitation

In the slower pace of the geriatric ward, Queenie began to make progress. Allowed plenty of time and with encouragement from the nursing, occupational therapy and physiotherapy staff, she became increasingly independent.

Domiciliary support following discharge:

home help

Meals on Wheels

Day Hospital

outside toilet therefore commode required

follow-up visit from geriatric liaison nurse

bed to be moved downstairs

Following discussion amongst the multidisciplinary team, a trial visit home with a ward nurse and an occupational therapist was arranged. A spinster at the age of 86, Queenie had outlived most of her closest friends and had no relatives. However, she was fortunate in having a good neighbour who was waiting at her door to welcome Queenie on her day's trial at home.

Following this visit, it was agreed that Queenie should be discharged home but that she would require extensive support.

Unfortunately, after only a month at home, Queenie's physical condition had deteriorated to such an extent that during a visit to the Day Hospital, her readmission to the Geriatric Unit was arranged.

REASSESSMENT

Once again, in the supportive environment of the rehabilitation ward, Queenie's condition improved. She had spent much of her time at home sitting in an armchair and had lost confidence in her own ability to cope. As she regained confidence, the question of her future was discussed once again by the multidisciplinary team.

Having had a private word with Queenie beforehand, the medical social worker suggested to the team that Queenie might settle well into a local authority old people's home.

Her name was added to the waiting list for a place.

RESIDENTIAL CARE

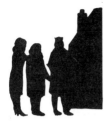

After several months of waiting, a place became available and Queenie consented to visit the home concerned 'just to have a look'. The visit also enabled the Officer-in-Charge of the home to assess whether she thought Queenie would be a suitable candidate to become a resident there.

Queenie was accompanied on her visit by the medical social worker and a nurse. On the way to the home, the medical social worker explained what a local authority home was.

Local authority residential care homes for the elderly: 'Part III' accommodation

Established as a requirement of Part III of the 1948 National Assistance Act which made it a statutory obligation for every local authority to provide residential accommodation for persons 'who by reason of age or infirmity are in need of care and attention which is not otherwise available to them'

Queenie was very surprised to find the home a modern, purpose-built one, not at all like some of the converted workhouses which are also used as residential homes. She enjoyed her visit, discovering that there were 50 residents in the home altogether, mainly women, and that most had their own rooms with a few sharing a double room.

Queenie was subsequently admitted to a ground floor room at the home. At that stage she could walk fairly well with a Zimmer frame and was continent provided she could get to the toilet fairly easily and in good time. Her rented terraced house was given up and the finality of this act led to a period of depression.

However, she was able to bring into the home some prized personal possessions which helped to stamp her individuality on her own room, and after the initial difficult settling-in period she adapted well to communal life.

Though rather forgetful she had a pleasant personality and enjoyed the company of staff and residents at the home.

LIVING IN PART III

Unfortunately, during the next few months Queenie's physical condition began to deteriorate and she became increasingly disorientated. At first the care staff were able to cope fairly well, prompting her to wash and dress and persuading her to participate in some of the activities in the home.

However, Queenie's increasing confusion, immobility and the onset of numerous episodes of urinary incontinence finally led to the Officer-in-Charge requesting that she be referred to the hospital Geriatric Unit again. The Consultant Geriatrician, having visited her in the home, agreed to admit her to his assessment ward.

RE-ADMISSION

Queenie was readmitted to the Geriatric Unit after almost a year in residential care. The sudden change in environment increased her disorientation and confusion further and the nursing staff found her difficult to manage.

Although she had become virtually wheelchair-bound, she now repeatedly attempted to stand and walk unaided, leading to a series of falls. A referral to the Consultant Psychogeriatrician confirmed the diagnosis of the early stages of *dementia*.

Dementia:

insidious onset
occurs more commonly in women than men
occurs most commonly in late 70s and 80s
Manifestations of dementia
forgetfulness, especially of recent events
neglect of personal hygiene

antisocial behaviour
failure to recognise relatives and friends
disorientation in time and place
incontinence
wandering behaviour

After a short period in the geriatric assessment ward, it was agreed that Queenie's disabilities had become so great that she should be transferred to the longstay geriatric ward.

Common reasons for admission to long-term care:

difficulty in walking
vertigo
falls
fainting attacks
mental impairment
stroke
cardiopulmonary problems
incontinence
Parkinsonism
decreased vision

Queenie's room at the local authority home was given up and her few prized possessions brought to the hospital. As soon as a bed became available in the continuing care ward, she was transferred.

CONTINUING CARE

During her initial period on the ward, the nursing staff found Queenie very unsettled. She slept badly, calling out during the night and disturbing other patients. She was covered in scratches and bruises from her many falls. Her appetite was poor and she remained incontinent of urine.

Having been thoroughly assessed medically, the nursing staff set about devising a care plan which would meet Queenie's individual nursing needs.

Despite her unsettled behaviour, no physical restraints at all were used. The nursing staff agreed that cotsides on the bed and 'geriatric'

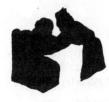

chairs with fixed tables would only serve to frustrate and anger Queenie, adding to her confusion.

All staff were asked to approach her quietly, to explain in detail anything that was about to happen, and to assist Queenie in her attempts to walk rather than trying to persuade her to sit down. The nursing staff soon discovered that Queenie disliked the noise of radio and television.

As Queenie became accustomed to her surroundings and familiar with the staff, her behaviour became less disruptive and noisy. It was agreed to formulate a plan to try and control her incontinence of urine and also to encourage her attempts to walk.

Continence training programme:

1 Commode by the bed at night
2 To sit within easy walking distance of the toilet during the day
3 To wear protective pants with disposable pad inserts during the day
4 Pattern of incontinence to be established by completing incontinence chart
5 To be assisted to the toilet/commode at regular intervals

A record of Queenie's progress on the continence training programme was charted, in order to establish the pattern of her incontinence over a 24 hour period. As the episodes of incontinence decreased, it became easier to involve Queenie in the activities of the ward.

Before long, Queenie's personality asserted itself in the lively atmosphere of the longstay ward despite her dementia. She became a great favourite of the Voluntary Services Coordinator whose job involved not only recruiting formal volunteers but also arranging services to be made available from the Red Cross and other local groups.

Queenie settled well into the ward, an individual whose dignity was respected despite the gradual disintegration of her personality.

Continence Chart

Week commencing _____ Name _____

PLEASE TICK IN GREY COLUMN EACH TIME URINE PASSED
PLEASE TICK IN WHITE COLUMN EACH TIME YOU ARE WET

	Mon		Tues		Wed		Thurs		Fri		Sat		Sun	
6 am														
7 am														
8 am														
9 am														
10 am														
11 am														
12 pm														
1 pm														
2 pm														
3 pm														
4 pm														
5 pm														
6 pm														
7 pm														
8 pm														
9 pm														
10 pm														
11 pm														
12 am														
1 am														
2 am														
3 am														
4 am														
5 am														
Totals														

Special instructions _____

What have you learnt about longstay care of the elderly from this chapter and what are your thoughts about it? Test yourself with these questions – your Tutor or Ward Sister may be interested in your views on longstay care.

1 What do you understand by the term 'Part III accommodation'? How is a patient in your hospital allocated a place in a Part III home? What training is available to Officers-in-Charge of Part III accommodation?

2 What are the main reasons for admission of elderly people to longstay care? What is the role of the Voluntary Services Co-ordinator in hospital? What programme of activities would you consider appropriate for a group of patients in a longstay ward on which you might be working?

3 Do you understand the meaning of 'reality orientation'? In the normal course of events during a day and night on your ward, how could you reinforce a programme of reality orientation with a confused elderly patient?

4 Why do you think the nursing staff in the preceding chapter did not favour the use of restraints such as cotsides and 'geriatric' chairs with fixed tables? What are your views on this?

**FURTHER
READING**

BROCKLEHURST, J. C. & KAMAL, A. 1983. *A Colour Atlas of Geriatric Medicine.* London: Wolfe Medical Publications Ltd.

DENHAM, M. J. (Ed). 1983. *Care of the Longstay Elderly Patient.* Beckenham, Kent: Croom Helm.

ELLIOTT, J. R. 1982. *Living in Hospital: the Social Needs of People in Long-Term Care.* 2nd ed. Oxford: Oxford University Press.

HOLDEN, U. P. & WOODS, R. T. 1982. *Reality Orientation – Psychological Approaches to the Confused Elderly.* Edinburgh: Churchill Livingstone.

NORMAN, A. J. 1980. *Rights and Risk – A discussion document on civil liberty in old age.* London: Centre for Policy on Ageing.

WHITTON, J. R. 1981. *Managing to Care in Homes for the Elderly.* Richmond, Surrey: Patten Press.

9 Care of the Dying

Mr Jefferies is a 75 year old widower admitted to the assessment ward of the Geriatric Unit from a private nursing home where he has been a resident for almost five years.

On admission to the ward he is given a thorough medical examination by the admitting doctor who confirms that Mr Jefferies is suffering from the later stages of *Parkinson's disease* and that he has developed *bronchopneumonia*. He requires terminal care.

Mr Jefferies is accompanied to the ward by one of the trained nurses from the private nursing home who knows him well. While planning his nursing care, the ward nurse is able to find out something of her new patient's past medical and social history. The more she is able to discover about her patient, the better able she will be to meet his needs.

Needs of the dying patient:

physical
psychological
spiritual
social

Mr Jefferies, already a widower at the age of 65, retired to a seaside resort on the west coast of England after a successful career as a bank manager. He had planned well for his retirement; the seaside town was very near the city where he had spent his working life, and many of his business friends had also chosen to retire to this area.

He moved into a bungalow within easy walking distance of local amenities such as shops and library, and which was well served by public transport. He enjoyed his own company and was fond of reading and tending his small garden.

His neighbours and acquaintances grew to know him as a pleasant but reserved man, who seemed to have adapted well to retirement, avoiding many of the common pitfalls.

As a bank manager, he had ensured that his financial status throughout retirement would remain more than adequate. He enjoyed the intellectual stimulation offered by his involvement with the University of the Third Age, and once a week he offered his services to a local voluntary group. He had also retained his involvement with the Pre-retirement Association of Great Britain.

University of the Third Age:

The aim of the University of the Third Age – or U3A for short – is to encourage older unemployed and retired people to find new interests and activities. No qualifications are needed for entry and no degrees, diplomas or certificates awarded. The first U3A in Great Britain was launched in Cambridge in 1981, and there is now a network throughout the country, each one developing to meet local needs.

Over a period of two or three years following his retirement, Mr Jefferies noticed an increasing tremor in his right hand when he was sitting reading. When he moved his hand to turn the page of his book or to pick up a cup, the tremor stopped. If he became excited or nervous it worsened.

He became particularly worried when he began to lose his balance for no apparent reason and finally agreed to visit his G.P. Suspecting a diagnosis of Parkinson's disease, Mr Jefferies' doctor arranged for him to see the Consultant Geriatrician in the Outpatients' Department of the local hospital.

The diagnosis was confirmed by the Geriatrician and a course of medication commenced.

Parkinson's disease (paralysis agitans):

A progressive, degenerative disease of the nervous system, affecting the basal ganglia of the cerebrum of the brain. First described as 'shaking palsy' in 1817 by a London doctor named James Parkinson.

cause:	unknown
onset:	insidious
affects:	more men than women
occurs:	in the latter half of life

Despite initial improvement as the medication took effect, the progressive nature of the disease began to take its toll and eventually after one of his follow-up visits to the Outpatients' Department, Mr Jefferies was admitted to the Geriatric Unit for assessment and a period of rehabilitation.

The Occupational Therapy and Physiotherapy Departments were particularly helpful in making available various aids to help him at home, his needs having been properly assessed following a home visit.

DISCHARGED HOME

For a period Mr Jefferies coped very well at home after his discharge, using to the full the aids which had been recommended. While in hospital he found he could walk well with a Rollator walking frame but it was of no use to him at home in the limited space of his bungalow. He also found the more conventional Zimmer frame cumbersome and tiring to lift.

Aids to daily living:

walking frame (if appropriate)
non-slip bath mat
bath and toilet 'grab rails'
raised toilet seat
non-slip table mats e.g. 'Dycem'
cutlery with 'built-up' handles e.g. 'Sunflower'

PROGRESSION OF THE DISEASE

The pattern of Mr Jefferies' Parkinsonism was characteristic. An intelligent man with a methodical, enquiring mind, he had found out as much as he could about his disease both from health care professionals and as a new member of the Parkinson's Disease Society. He knew what to expect.

Clinical features of Parkinsonism:

hypokinesia: diminished power of movement
              tremor
              muscular rigidity

characterised by:

mask-like, unblinking facial expression; shuffling, hurried (festinate) gait; stooping posture; dysphagia and alimentary tract problems; inertia; micrographia; slurred speech; mental disturbance; dementia; incontinence.

PLANNING AHEAD

Concerned for his future as a widower living alone without close relatives or friends, Mr Jefferies decided that he would make enquiries about selling his bungalow and moving permanently into a private home. In view of the progressive nature of his illness he opted for a nursing home rather than a residential care home.

Several nursing homes were mentioned to him by the community nursing staff and he arranged to visit some. Finally he chose a small establishment which offered him a large, single, ground floor room with a separate communal lounge. With the proceeds of the sale of his bungalow and his nest-egg of 'rainy day' savings he was content that he would be able to continue to meet the fees.

At the age of 70, after only 5 years of independent retirement, Mr Jefferies moved into the private nursing home with a few small items of furniture, many books and some small treasured personal possessions.

LIFE IN THE NURSING HOME

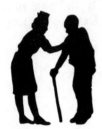

As the years passed Mr Jefferies began to require more and more help from the team of trained nurses and their untrained nursing assistants. He found it particularly difficult to turn over in bed, to get into a sitting position when he had been lying down, and to stand up and start walking when he had been sitting.

The difficulty caused at mealtimes by his hand tremors made him embarrassed and distressed and he took all his meals in his room. He began to need help with washing and dressing, particularly as the fine finger movements required to do up his buttons became impossible.

Almost imperceptibly, his dependence increased and he became more and more frail. Finally, with the onset of bronchopneumonia the nursing team agreed that Mr Jefferies' needs were too great to be met by the limited resources available in the small nursing home. His admission to hospital was arranged by the visiting G.P.

TERMINAL CARE

Bronchopneumonia:

a common disease of old age

predisposing factors:
immobility
dysphagia
cardiac failure
upper respiratory tract infections
chronic bronchitis

The nurse responsible for admitting Mr Jefferies to the ward and planning his care is now better able to appreciate the type of life he has led and the difficulties imposed upon him by the limitations of his disease. In planning his nursing care she takes into account the effects of both the long-standing illness and the bronchopneumonia, which is not being treated with antibiotics.

PHYSICAL NEEDS

The smallest detail of physical nursing care takes on added importance when caring for the dying patient. Mr Jefferies is nursed in bed on a sheepskin underblanket with a bed cradle in place to keep the weight of the bedclothes off his legs. His skin is very dry and he is at considerable risk from developing pressure sores. The decision to insert an indwelling urinary catheter is taken to maintain his comfort and hygiene in view of intransigent urinary incontinence.

Mr Jefferies' position is changed regularly; he is sweating profusely, requiring frequent gentle washes and fresh bed linen. His mouth is very dry and he is not able to eat or drink. However, he appreciates the opportunity to suck some flavoured crushed ice. A soothing cream applied to his lips prevents them from cracking.

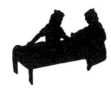

The nurses speak gently to Mr Jefferies as they tend to him, continuing to address him courteously by name even though he is not able to communicate with them.

As Mr Jefferies' condition deteriorates, it becomes increasingly important to position him in such a way that he is able to breathe comfortably. The nursing staff are aware that if his chest becomes very congested and sounds 'bubbly', an injection of hyoscine can be prescribed which will dry the secretions.

OTHER NEEDS

In meeting Mr Jefferies' physical needs, the nurses also take into account his emotional, spiritual and social needs. As he has always been accustomed to the privacy of a single room and his own company, it is agreed that he will be more peaceful and comfortable in a room on his own.

However, nurses pause frequently to speak to him when they are not tending his physical needs, and from time to time a nurse sits quietly with him, holding his hand.

Although he has not been particularly active as a church goer, his religion is ascertained and the relevant minister visits. Several of his friends and some of the staff of the nursing home also spend time sitting talking quietly to him. A framed photograph of his wife is brought to his room and placed where he can see it easily.

After only two days in hospital, Jasper Jefferies died peacefully with a friend at his side.

TEST YOURSELF

Can you answer the following questions? Ask your Tutor or Ward Sister for help if you get into difficulties.

1 What advice could you give to someone about to retire on how to plan for an active and fulfilled retirement? What pitfalls might you warn them about?

2 What are the principal features of Parkinson's disease? What other factors can precipitate the symptoms of Parkinsonism? What measures apart from medication can be used to treat Parkinson's disease?

3 Have you ever visited a hospice specialising in the care of terminally ill patients? Do you think this is a good system of care? Why?

4 What is the procedure for resuscitation of the patients in the department of geriatric medicine in which you work? Do you agree with this procedure and the philosophy behind it?

FURTHER READING

ISSACS, B. (Ed). 1981. *Recent Advances in Geriatric Medicine No. 2.* Edinburgh: Churchill Livingstone.

KUBLER-ROSS, E. 1982. *Living with Death and Dying.* London: Souvenir Press.

LAMERTON, R. 1980. *Care of the Dying.* Harmondsworth, Middx: Pelican Books.

MIDWINTER, E. 1982. *Age is Opportunity: Education and Older People.* London: Centre for Policy on Ageing.

ROBBINS, J. 1983. *Caring for the Dying Patient and the Family.* London: Harper and Row.

STORRS, A. 1984. *Geriatric Nursing.* 3rd ed. Nurses' Aids Series. Eastbourne, Sussex: Baillière Tindall.

10 Conclusion

Better health care of the general population has meant that fewer young patients are to be found in hospital. With the exception of maternity and paediatric wards, elderly people now tend to be in the majority in every hospital ward.

As Departments of Geriatric Medicine have developed, the original admitting age of 65 has tended to increase in line with the increasing age of the population generally.

The overall effect of this trend is that non-specialist wards are beginning to cater more and more for the 'young' old. Many specialised Geriatric Units are beginning to quote 70 or even 75 as the 'minimum qualifying age' for admission – the 'old' old.

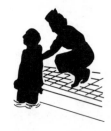

Aggressive rehabilitation programmes and emphasis on care in the community mean a much higher proportion of elderly clients on the caseloads of community workers, a greater reliance on voluntary services, and a greater need than ever for support for the network of informal carers.

It is the responsibility of every health care professional to be aware of the special needs of the elderly, bearing in mind that the term 'elderly' refers to people whose ages range across four decades of life.

It is the specialist's responsibility to recognise the urgent need for collaboration. The care of the elderly cannot be undertaken in isolation.

It is every individual's responsibility to examine their own attitudes to ageing. Positive planning to meet future needs will only happen with the development of positive attitudes.

Health Education

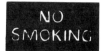

Leaving preparation for a healthy old age until retirement is too late. Looking after health throughout life is a good insurance for a healthy old age.

There is a general tacit acceptance that retirement means the end of active life; having 'earned a good rest', you can slow down and stop. In fact the more active people are after retirement, the fitter and healthier they will be.

There is too much acceptance of illness as a result of ageing – 'What can you expect at your age?' – whereas in fact many trivial ailments can be treated and cured.

At the same time, encouraging elderly people to be more positive in their own attitudes to health has to be matched by an equal commitment from health care professionals – and by adequate resources.

Preparation for retirement

The majority of people have retirement thrust upon them, sometimes unwillingly. The advantage of knowing your full-time working life is to cease abruptly at a specific time is that you can plan in advance to cope with it.

Some companies offer pre-retirement classes to advise on how to avoid the pitfalls and make the most of the pleasures. Sometimes it is possible to withdraw from work gradually, changing from full-time to part-time work before retirement. Involvement with the Pre-retirement Association can be helpful.

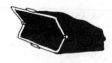

Unquestionably, very many people are adversely affected by a drastic reduction in income which cannot be altogether offset by careful planning and which will colour the way in which they are obliged to live their lives. Voluntary agencies such as Age Concern are vociferous in encouraging the elderly to claim all the statutory benefits to which they are entitled.

Voluntary Organisations

The number of voluntary organisations involved in some way with the elderly is vast. Some provide financial assistance, some provide practical support, occasionally in conjunction with statutory agencies, and some are very active politically in attempting to influence attitudes towards, and provisions for, the elderly. Some agencies manage to combine several of these roles very successfully.

The days of the 'flower hat brigade' are long gone. Most voluntary organisations are well-organised and efficient. Without doubt, the involvement of the voluntary sector is now recognised as essential in 'propping up' statutory services in many respects.

Aspects of Institutionalised Care

When a Department of Geriatric Medicine is functioning effectively it offers a service to the elderly which is second to none.

Nevertheless, despite many years of claiming that services for the elderly are a priority, too many Departments of Geriatric Medicine are still housed in hopelessly inadequate, outdated buildings.

Many practical nursing problems have been identified as being associated with the fact that four-fifths of geriatric hospitals are adapted premises (Norton, 1967). While some wards may have been upgraded, critical shortages in toilet, bath and dayroom areas are often highlighted (Wells, 1980).

Research has indicated that reducing the number of beds per ward may be the only way to provide the fundamental priority of the minimum standard bed area which is essential to any equipment and furniture improvement programme (Wells, 1980).

Staffing

Poor recruitment of trained nurses has led to inadequate teaching and supervision of learner nurses and auxiliaries. Wells (1980) said that 'auxiliary nurses, the most numerous caregivers for the hospitalised elderly, had little or no idea of the cause and care of common problems in the elderly'.

The same might still be said of some health care professionals, ignorant of the multifaceted nursing problems of the elderly, who believe that adequate 'basic nursing care' can be delivered by untrained personnel.

The fact that all nurses in training are now required to undergo practical experience in the care of the elderly bodes well for the future of the specialty. All tutors and all nurse managers involved with the care of the elderly in the future will at least have experienced the specialty at first hand.

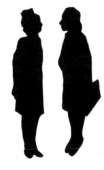

Care of the elderly is not confined to geriatric wards, of course, and some Health Authorities have recognised the need to disseminate specialist information to non-specialist wards by the appointment of Nurse Consultants in the care of the elderly who are available to advise in every ward on the skills of geriatric nursing.

Specialist nurses working as Continence Advisers are having a growing impact on the promotion of continence in the elderly. The acceptance of incontinence as inevitable and irreversible is very gradually breaking down in the face of their very positive and aggressive approach.

As the number of Community Psychiatric Nurses with a special interest in the care of the elderly increases, so a more positive attitude to coping with elderly mentally infirm people in the community will develop.

Residential Care

There is a growing interest in the care of the elderly in local authority and private residential care homes, and in private nursing homes. As legislation attempts to tighten control over the rapidly growing private sector, problems are increasing in the public sector.

There is no statutory requirement that the Officers-in-Charge of local authority homes should have any kind of nursing qualification, despite the fact that residents are becoming increasingly dependent as their average age increases. At the moment, if residents require any professional nursing, it must be provided by the already overstretched community nursing services.

National Health Service Nursing Homes

In 1980, a Government White Paper (Growing Older) suggested that nursing homes for the elderly within the framework of the National Health Service was a feasible possibility.

As various pilot schemes were put into operation, a major objective for these homes was defined as providing a homely environment for heavily dependent elderly patients who would otherwise require care in a long-term hospital ward.

The move away from longstay care in institutions is to be welcomed. Creating a cosy atmosphere in a barn-like dormitory of 20 or (more usually) nearly 30 beds is a daunting task.

Giving residents their own rooms where they can retain at least some of their own possessions begins to make sense of a philosophy of 'homely' care where the dignity of the individual is respected.

Collaboration

The incidence of mental infirmity increases with age, and therefore the predicted growth in the proportion of very elderly people in the population is accompanied by an increase in the number of mentally frail old people.

As well as the creation of units specifically designed for this type of patient, alongside the development of specialist Departments of Psychiatry for the Elderly (as recommended in the document, *The Rising Tide*), there are also some joint assessment wards where beds are available for both psychiatric and geriatric consultants to admit patients.

Similarly, orthopaedic and geriatric consultants sometimes share their expertise in joint wards, removing the necessity to transfer patients physically from one ward to another as their need for specialist care changes from one consultant to the other.

Community Care

In principle, everyone welcomes the shift away from institution to community. However, this must be seen in realistic terms. Rehabilitating a patient for discharge home has to take into account an enormous number of factors.

'Home' could mean the tenth floor of a high-rise block of flats with the lift frequently out of order. If Meals on Wheels are only available for 3 days a week, who will buy the food to cook on the remaining 4 days?

Home helps are able to do limited cleaning, but nothing very extensive – certainly not washing sheets or heavy cleaning.

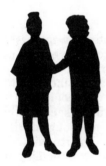

The problems encountered by the nurses in the primary health care team need to be appreciated by nurses in hospital – and vice versa. While the appointment of a Geriatric Liaison Nurse who can see both sides of the coin goes some way to breaking down communication barriers, a future where training made the roles of hospital and community nurses in the geriatric specialty interchangeable would certainly help to ease the problems even further.

The Future and Elderly People

New challenges in the care of elderly people become apparent all the time – the growth in the number of black and Asian old people in Britain is one which is currently under examination.

However, the fact is that most elderly people are fit and well and living fulfilled, active lives just like everybody else – in every respect.

For a good many years, policies which affect their care because of their age have been in-

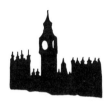

flicted upon them. Their own knowledge and experience have been underestimated and underused.

There is a growing awareness that they themselves can influence policies. The passivity of the past is being replaced by positive action – the American 'Grey Panthers' have proved that elderly people have a tremendous amount of potential as a powerful political influence.

Local Pensioners' Action Groups are spreading like wildfire in this country. More than any other development, that could be the greatest hope for the future of the care of the elderly.

FURTHER READING

NORTON, D. 1967. *Hospitals of the Longstay Patient.* Oxford: Pergamon Press.

WELLS, T. J. 1980. *Problems in Geriatric Nursing Care: A study of Nurses' Problems in Care of Old People in Hospitals.* Edinburgh: Churchill Livingstone.

DHSS/Scottish Office/Welsh Office/Northern Ireland Office. 1981. *Growing Older.* London: Her Majesty's Stationery Office.

NHS HEALTH ADVISORY SERVICE. 1982. *The Rising Tide – Developing Services for Mental Illness in Old Age.* NHS Health Advisory Service.

USEFUL NAMES AND ADDRESSES

Age Concern (England)
Bernard Sunley House,
60 Pitcairn Road,
Mitcham
Surrey

Age Concern (Northern Ireland)
128 Great Victoria Street,
Belfast 2
BT2 7BG

Age Concern (Scotland)
33 Castle Street,
Edinburgh
EH2 3DN

Age Concern (Wales)
1 Park Grove,
Cardiff
CF1 3BJ

Alzheimer's Disease Society,
3rd Floor,
Bank Buildings,
Fulham Broadway,
London
SW6 1EP

The Arthritis and Rheumatism
Council,
41 Eagle Street,
London
WC1R 4AR

Association of Carers,
Medway Homes,
Balfour Road,
Rochester,
Kent
ME4 6QU

Association of Continence
Advisers,
The Disabled Living Foundation,
346 Kensington High Street,
London
W14 8NS

British Association for Service to
the Elderly,
3 Keele Farmhouse,
Keele,
Newcastle-under-Lyme,
Staffs
ST5 5AR

British Diabetic Association,
10 Queen Anne Street,
London
W1M 0BD

British Journal of Geriatric
Nursing,
Baillière Tindall,
1 Vincent Square,
London
SW1P 2PN

British Red Cross Society,
9 Grosvenor Crescent,
London
SW1X 7EJ

The Centre for Policy on Ageing,
Nuffield Lodge,
Regent's Park,
London
NW1 4RS

The Chest, Heart and Stroke
Association,
Tavistock House North,
Tavistock Square,
London
WC1H 9JE

Counsel and Care for the Elderly,
131 Middlesex Street,
London
E1 7JF

Crossroads Care Attendant
Scheme Trust,
11 Whitehall Road,
Rugby,
Warwickshire
CV21 3AQ

CRUSE,
126 Sheen Road,
Richmond,
Surrey

Help the Aged,
32 Dover Street,
London
W1A 2AP

The Health Education Council,
78 New Oxford Street,
London
WC1A 1AH

King's Fund Centre,
126 Albert Street,
London
NW1 7NF

MIND (National Association for
Mental Health)
22 Harley Street,
London
W1N 2ED

National Council for Carers and
Their Dependants,
29 Chilworth Mews,
London
W2 3RG

Parkinson's Disease Society,
3 Portland Place,
London
W1N 3DG

Royal Association for Disability
and Rehabilitation (RADAR),
25 Mortimer Street,
London
W1N 8AB

Royal National Institute for the
Blind,
224 Great Portland Street,
London
W1N 6AA

Royal National Institute for the
Deaf,
105 Gower Street,
London
WC1E 6AH

RCN Society of Geriatric
Nursing,
Royal College of Nursing,
20 Cavendish Square,
London
W1M 0AB

The Pre-retirement Association
of Great Britain and Northern
Ireland,
19 Undine Street,
Tooting,
London
SW17 8PP

University of the Third Age,
6 Parkside Gardens,
London
SW19 5EY

Women's Royal Voluntary
Service,
17 Old Park Lane,
London
W1Y 4AJ

INDEX